One Day at a Time,
with Guillain-Barré Syndrome, and CIDP

By
Michael J. Kiser

Edited by
LK Kelley

Published by DragonEye Publishing

One Day at a Time With Guillain-Barré Syndrome & CIDP
Copyright © 2018. By Michael Kiser

Publisher info. Contact
DragonEye Publishing
753A Linden Pl.
Elmira, New York, 14901

For Questions Phone: 1-(607)-333-5256

For information about our books, and for special discounts for single / bulk purchases, please contact DragonEye Publishing Ordering Dept. at:
Website: DragonEyePublishers.com
Email: Orders@DragonEyePublishers.com

To request one of our authors for speaking engagements or book signings, please contact DragonEye Publishing Publicity Dept. at:
Directors@DragonEyePublishers.com

Published by
DragonEye Publishing

ISBN 13: 978-1-61500-224-5   (Paperback)
ISBN 13: 978-1-61500-225-2   (EBook)

Library of Congress Control Number: 2019902263

DragonEye Publishing, First Edition: March 23, 2019
First Printing: March 23, 2019

10 9 8 7 6 5 4 3 2 1

Manufactured in the United States of America

Contents

Preface

All of our life, we take our body and our immune system for granted. We think it will keep us all healthy, as long as we take care of our body and our health. But, no matter how well we take care of these, it is impossible to know if, or when, our immune system might break down, even if one is completely healthy.

My immune system reversed from healing my body to attacking the very core of my body's function, nervous system, and muscles. Without normal function, our body totally shuts down, and it may even cause death.

The name of this illness is called "Guillain Barre Syndrome / Acute Relapsing Chronic Inflammatory Demyelinating Polyneuropathy". By telling my own story, I hope this will help people understand what someone goes through during this immune system syndrome. This book is also for those who might unfortunately end up experiencing this type of syndrome, since there is little known about why it comes about.

I had talked to people that had this syndrome years ago, who said that after the immune system fully recovers from the attack on the body, it will return to the way it was before this attack occurred, or at least very near to the way it was before the attack occurred. That is about 90%-95%, and it also depends on each person. Since we are all different, there is always a possibility that our bodies might not reach 100% normal. You might have some weak muscles in the feet, legs, and arms, which will remain for some time, after the body has almost or totally recovered from Guillain Barre Syndrome. If the treatment works on reversing your immune system, you will begin to notice almost immediately. But the healing of the nerves will take months to years, depending on how much damage is done. This is a time of not knowing personally how much damage has been done to the nerves themselves, and how long it will take them to heal. From what I have learned from my neurologist, it takes a healthy nerve a month to heal one inch depending on the damage. From my personal experience, I can say that while it may be hard, it is very important to keep track of the healing process of your nerves and not to worry too much about your muscles. Your nerves are very important. It is up to the individual person, who is experiencing this syndrome, to monitor what you are feeling in your nerves since there is no way for the doctors to know or feel what you are sensing. Only you know how the nerves are healing. Keep in mind this is not a fast healing process. It is the slowest healing that you might ever come to experience in your life. One day all of your nerves that were damaged from this syndrome will heal completely. When that time will come is all unknown, but it will come.

Chapter
1

A Healthy Life

I am Michael J. Kiser and this is my true life-changing story. I was born in Elmira, New York in 1966. I was healthy and active my whole life. At the age of thirteen, I was active in sports at Ernie Davis Junior High School, and I was involved in soccer for two years. I was in an archery league in Pine City, New York, for two years. After entering into high school, at Elmira Free Academy (EFA) from 1981-1985, I was involved in bowling, very active in running, and distant bike cycling with a few of my friends.

After high school in 1985, I had a chance to go to film school in New York City. This was my goal all the way through high school. I majored in art, photography, ceramics, sculpturing figures, TV broadcasting, and script writing. Therefore, my parents paid for the film home school class during the summer of 1985, so that I could start the fall film classes in October of 1985. After a month, I decided to change my direction and stopped the summer home course. As I look back today, I wish that I had completed the course.

As the fall of 1985 arrived, I started working with Manpower (a job finder). I worked several short-term jobs, and two jobs in factories. One job was at Elmira Heat Treating, where they treated metal parts of all sorts, for many manufacturers. I worked there until the end of 1987. Next, I worked at Toshiba-Westinghouse in the high voltage /aging department until the summer of 1989, where Cathode Ray Tubes (CRT's) are made, which are the TV tubes for television and computer screens.

In the summer of 1987, I began writing a book about my understanding of the spiritual growth of evolution. I sent it to a few publishers in 1988 and 1989. Only one was interested in the book. The interested publisher would have published my book, if I paid them $9,000. At that time I did not have the money.

In the summer of 1988, my ex-fiancé introduced me to Cindy Green, who was one of her girlfriends. They both went to Elmira Southside High School and started college together. At that time, I had been working for two years at Toshiba Westinghouse Manufacturing. Since I was there for some time, I was able to have two weeks of vacation. Just before the start of my vacation, I finally met Cindy. Then after knowing her for only a week, I asked Cindy if she would like to take a vacation with me, she decided to join me. We went to the Black Canyon of Gunnison in Western Colorado, spending a week camping and hiking in the canyon.

I was still working at Toshiba-Westinghouse in the spring of 1989. I became sick from working in the High Voltage / Aging department for the CRT's, so I had to quit and take a couple of months to get better.

At this time, Cindy and I began work at Long John Silver's restaurant in Horseheads, New York. It was new, and we worked from the opening until the summer of May 1990, when we decided to get married and leave Painted Post, New York.

Cindy and I moved to Denver, Colorado, after we were married. After we were settled into an apartment, we both found retail jobs in different locations in the Denver and Aurora area. After being in Colorado for a couple of months, we became involved in cliff climbing, mountain hiking, and mountain camping. We enjoyed driving up to the mountains of the Continental Divide. We went every spare moment we had to go together or by ourselves to explore the uniqueness the mountains had to offer.

In September of 1990, we heard about a group of people that met with common interests of the UFO phenomenon. I was very interested in UFO's, and wanted to see what they knew and had to offer as far as information. So, Cindy and I made plans to go to one of their meetings. We were impressed, and joined the group, becoming board members.

At this time, Cindy and I decided it was time for us to start our project. Therefore, in December of 1990, we created our own magazine called "In Search of the Universal Truth". Within the magazine, we delved into the spiritual questions of life. We asked others these questions to see if they might have any answers or insight to the many questions that we all ponder, including all of the seen and unseen worlds that are all around us. Regardless of our beliefs and those from our families, partners and friends, our magazine questioned other beliefs. Off-world beings, have been visiting different human civilizations, since the beginning of time, if not before time itself. This led us to believe that the information that we received could be the next step in the evolution of man. It also included the coming Mayan Calendar apocalypse of December 21, 2012, as well as other ideas.

On July 2, 1993, after living in Colorado for 3 years, Cindy passed away, and I had her flown back to Elmira, New York. After her funeral, I stayed there for two weeks visiting our families and friends, and then I returned to Denver to continue my life. I continued with the projects that Cindy and I had been doing together, before her passing.

After Cindy's death, I spent a few days by myself as I remembered the love we shared and the experiences that Cindy and I had during our five years together. I will never forget her. Just as I will never forget all the people that were a part of my life, and the ladies that I would come to be married to during my life here on Earth.

It was at this time, I began another relationship with a friend of ours named Judy. We had known each other since late October of 1990.

Judy and I began our relationship, during the second week of July, soon after Cindy had passed away. In the second week of August 1993, Judy told me that she was pregnant, and we were both happy to be having a child.

However, in late September of 1993 Judy changed. She wanted me out of her home and her life by the end of October 1993. As the time came for me to leave, Judy did not apologize for either her actions or word.

Time passed, and I left messages for Judy, but she did not return them. Even though I went to her home, she still did not open her door to speak to me. February 1994 arrived, and Judy finally called me at work to ask if we could get together to talk about us as a family. We met, and spoke about becoming a family, which led to the two of us moving in together, again, but she decided there could not be a relationship between us.

On May 4, 1994 our son, Jonathan, was born. Judy only wanted me to be there for Jonathan. No matter what happened, I was always going to be around for my son. But, Judy just didn't want a family. At the end of May 1997, Judy repeated her actions in October of 1993, and threatened to call the police. Therefore, I gathered up some clothes, and Judy's brother, Glenn Volmer, who had shown up, took me to a hotel.

When Jonathan was five years old, Judy, Jonathan and I began camping and hiking together in the mountains. She still didn't want to be in a relationship, but we continued to do things together until 2002.

I worked for K Mart from 1994 through 2001, and then, a security company in the fall of 2001, two months before K Mart filed for chapter 13. I had been there for a long time, and had just received a promotion to management. Since I was the last one to be promoted into the management position, I was the first to let go. At the same time, I was also working the graveyard shift as a security officer from the late summer of 2001.

The years passed and by late 2002, Judy no longer joined us, and our Father and Son outings only included Jonathan and me. Between 2001 through 2005, I worked for four Security Companies, and on my days off, Jonathan and I "did our own thing" as father and son. We did many things such as hiking and camping in the mountains.

The spring of 2005 found me being asked to work a lot of overtime. I had saved up some money, and I saw my chance to publish my writings, that I been writing, since 1987. Eventually, I started my own book publishing company in April of 2005.

By the fall of 2005, I was still working for a security company, and Judy wanted more money in addition to what I had been paying to her for child support. I could not really afford to pay her more, but I did. At the same time I was telling Judy that if I kept giving her the additional money, I would not be able to afford to pay my bills or rent. Judy did not care as long as she received more money. So, I paid her even more money. I eventually was evicted from my home, and even though she did not like the idea of me living in her home, Judy let me stay with her, since the reason for my being evicted was because of her demands.

From the fall of 2005 until February 2006, I lived with Judy and our son Jonathan. I was working through Labor Ready Services, which is a day labor service. In February of 2006, Judy decided she did not want me staying at her home. I moved out to live in a motel, until the summer of 2006, when I found a place to stay as a roommate.

Chapter
2

Warning Signs

I had been a healthy and active man for 40 years.

We all think that since we are healthy and active, we will remain that way, if we do everything required in maintaining our body's health. We all think, "if I treat my body well and keep healthy, my body will return the same to me". However, our bodies are very complex, and we just do not know what might happen, especially when we take our bodies for granted.

On May 1, 2006, I had worked as a groundskeeper for a housing complex in Parker, Colorado for just over a month. One day, I stepped on a sprinkler box lid cover. Part of the lid corner was broken, and the lid teeter tottered, causing me to lose my balance. My left foot was on the cover and fell into a one-foot deep hole, where the sprinkler controls are. I was not thinking about this happening. However, I continued working throughout that day and afterward, for several days.

Then on May 14, 2006, as the workday ended, something started to affect my body. It started with both feet and hands at the same time, becoming numb and tingled. The sensation did not stop. The tingling continued in both hands and feet, so I made sure to drink lots of water, because the day was in the high 90's. I thought if I drank plenty of water, this feeling would end. When the day ended, I went home and rested, but the feeling continued for the rest of the night. I thought it might have been just from the hot day and the hot air, and I continued to drink plenty of water all night.

When I awoke the next day to dress for work, I noticed that the feelings were still present in both my feet and hands. Because we are taught to believe that our bodies are equipped to heal us, I continued being positive. So, I just let my body deal with what it was going through and believe that it would heal on its own.

A week later, it had not changed, but suddenly, it was different. Trying to describe it is a bit hard. But, it is the feeling one gets, when you hit your funny bone, and it almost takes away your breath from the shock..

During this time, I continued doing things with Jonathan. We played ball and ran around chasing each other, just like the things that a father and their 12-year-old child do.

It had been two weeks at the end of May, this feeling was still with me. The numbness and tingling had moved up my legs to both knees and into my hands. If climbed upward, progressing into both of my forearms. So, I started to do some more stretching for my neck, spine, and shoulder, along with my waist just in case I had a vertebra pinching a nerve that might be causing the feelings that had continued for the previous three weeks.

After dealing with these feelings day-in and day-out for a month, the numbness and the tingling had worked its way up my legs and arms.

I was living in a hotel room for about 3 months, at this point. One of the ladies that I worked with on that property, mentioned that her friend lived across the street from her. He had a two-bedroom home, and he was interested in having a roommate. I made plans to meet with this young man. After we met, I resided there from the end of May through June 28, 2006.

Judy knew about my problems, and suggested that I start drinking a tea called Hawthorn, that is purported to heal the nerves from nerve damage. Jonathan and I also started using a form of healing that is called Reiki Healing. Judy and I had been Reiki Healers, since 1993, and Jonathan has been a Reiki healer since 1995.

Jonathan began working on the bottom of my feet, and I worked on the healing at my waist in an attempt to keep this from evolving any further than it already had and to help the healing process.

Chapter
3

Reiki Healing

Reiki Healing is a 2,500-year-old Chinese technique of natural healing. Energy from the universe enters into the body through the top of our head, the energy is expelled out through the palms of our hands. The practice is quite easy. Place your hands on the other person where healing is needed. Both will feel the heat (energy), flowing from the person performing the healing, into the area where the hands have contact on the one who is ill. The purpose of this type of healing is to help realign the energies in the body where the area's normal energy patterns have been disrupted.

I refused to let these feelings keep me from enjoying the time with my son, Jonathan.

As the second week of June 2006 arrived, Jonathan and I headed to the mountains to hopefully divert my attention. At that time, I had no idea what was going on with my body, or how long it would go on.

Despite what I was experiencing, I was not going to let it interfere with spending time or doing things with our son. That included walking in the mountains, even though it was very difficult to be active.

We had not been to the mountains in a while, so we decided to head to Devils Head in Colorado to spend some time together. This was Jonathan's first time to Devils Head, and my fourth. I knew that walking to the mountain's peak would be involved.

I had a feeling that this time with Jonathan would be the last time for us to spend a weekend together, so I wanted to enjoy it. When we arrived at our destination, I grabbed my pack with our drinks and food, and we made our way to the trail for the hour-long walk to the peak of Devils Head. I found that I needed to take several short rests, during the walk to the top, because of the numbness, tingling, and the weakening in both of my feet and legs. I had done this walk three times over the past three years and each time I had done it non-stop. I had walked this same trail in about thirty-five minutes prior to this. Nevertheless, Jonathan and I made it to the base of the peak, where we found a spot for a late afternoon lunch, and to make sure we re-hydrated with juice and water, before we continued to the peak. After we finished with our lunch and rested for a little bit longer, we continued to the peak of Devils Head to the forest service fire watchtower.

As Jonathan and I start walking up the eighty plus steps to the top to the watchtower, I had to take several breaks, walking was bothering my legs. I was not going to quit so we rested a bit, before we continued to the peak. After about fifteen minutes, we arrived, and the view was magnificent. The weather was nice and the sky was clear for about a couple hundred miles in all directions. We stayed at the watchtower for about a half hour, gazing out at the plains to the east and the mountain ranges that run north and south. We turned our eyes to the west upon the width of the mountain ranges. After about a half hour, we descended to the base of the peak.

As we walked around to the south side, Jonathan found a trail that wound to the south side.

Jonathan asked, "Dad have you walked this trail that goes this way?"

"No I always have taken the north trail, which is the one that we walked up here on... Do you want to take that trail?" I replied to Jonathan.

"Only if you are up to it dad."

"We can take that trail... You can lead the way." Jonathan said.

"Okay then... I say we take this trail." I replied. "I am right behind you Jonathan."

The trail began to disappear after about fifteen minutes.

"Dad the trail stops here."

"Well... Let me take a look...."

I made my way stepping over fallen trees and around the shrubs to where Jonathan was standing at the end of the trail.

"Well, I guess the trail stops here, I think. What do you think Jonathan? Do you want to go back and retrace our steps walking to the peak?"

Jonathan said, "No. I still want to go this way. We have to find the trail."

"Okay then we will continue. Where do you think the trail is? Which way do you think we should go?" I pointed in a direction. "What about this way. We might find the trail over there."   Jonathan agreed.

"Yeah. Let's go that way, and see if we can find the trail again."

A few minutes later, we came to a trail.

"Dad, I think I found the trail again."

"That's great, Jonathan."

But, the trail ended once again.

Jonathan yelled at me.

"Dad… You will not believe what happened."

I yelled back.

"What happened?"

"The trail ended again!"

"Okay. Let's take a break, and I will be there in a minute."

"Okay. I'll wait for you on a fallen tree that's by me."

I caught up to him, and we sat looking around. There were some rocks that were stacked on top of each other scattered all over the place.

"What do you think about those rocks, Jonathan?"

"I think that we should follow them. Maybe they make up several trails." He waved his hand. "See? Some of them go this way, and those over there go in the other direction."

Jonathan continued to lead the way around the east side Devils Head Peak, and there, the trail was covered with rocks and downed trees, making it very difficult for me to walk, but I managed to make it with the help of Jonathan.

Forty minutes later, we finally arrived at the connection to the north side of the trail that led to the base of Devils Head. At the junction of these two trails, Jonathan and I sat on a bench, and rested. We pulled out some snacks and bottles of water to drink, before continuing down the mountain trail to where we had parked the car.

In June of 2006, I was finding it harder to work, walk, sit, and even to hold onto things. I had been enjoying my life and my son. Jonathan was still see-sawing back and forth between Judy and me. I was becoming harder for Jonathan, as he watched me become unable to do the things that we both had enjoyed doing together.

I did not associate the feeling that I was experiencing to the hole that I had tripped into a month earlier. But, I began to wonder if it could have been related in one form or another. Maybe it had caused a nerve to become pinched. I was still stretching my waist, spine, neck, and shoulders for this whole month and it wasn't helping.

I continued to work, but I was still continuing to experience the weakness, numbness, and tingling in both my feet and hands. It was now moving further up my legs and arms, and becoming difficult for me to work. Walking became more difficult, now, because it was moving toward my waist. It was affecting my vision as well. I was experiencing sporadic side-by-side double vision.

I went to a chiropractor who dealt with spine realignment. Hoping that he might be able to help. He took two x-rays of my neck, spine, and waist. After he adjusted my neck, and the double vision was gone. However, everything else was still present and I was not getting any better, but I was getting much worse.

By the end of June, I was losing my balance, and had begun falling down. Jonathan supplied his shoulder for balance, as all the muscles in both legs became too weak. If I turned just right, or if my feet did not lift up to take the next step I would fall down.

I became worse as each day passed. My feet began to swell to a point. My ankles lost the strength to hold my feet still as I tried to put on my shoes. The strength in my hands and wrists was also gone. It was so hard to hold onto things like a glass or even the silverware when I ate. I finally started to worry, and knew that this was also hard on Jonathan. Just seeing his dad having a hard time doing ordinary things with him and not being able to play or have fun together hurt.

Chapter
4

Hospitalized for Treatment

June 28, 2006

I finally decided it was time to seek out medical assistance. I headed to Rose Medical Center in Denver, Colorado, where I was in the emergency room for four hours. The emergency room physician contacted a special, neurological doctor. It was decided that I be admitted after tests were run. They would try to stop the progression, and see if there was a way to reverse what was transpiring. I hoped that the answer could be found.

Since I had only about ten percent use of my leg muscles, I could not feel my feet, and had no balance at all, I was informed by the nurse on arriving to my room, that I would need to call the CNA for assistance to the bathroom. After the CNA left the room, I called Judy to inform both her and Jonathan know what was going on, and that I had been admitted into the hospital. I had no idea how long I would be there.

That first night, about twelve tests were scheduled. An MRI was up first to see if there might be a tumor, or if I had, had a stroke without knowing it. Blood work was ordered as well as a spinal tap to check on the cerebrospinal fluid that bathes the spinal cord, along with tests on my brain and my protein. In addition, a Nerve Conduction Velocity (NCV) was also ordered.

June 29, 2006

After my breakfast, a male CNA came into my room to help me into a wheelchair, and then he wheeled me to a room for the NCV test, which measured how long it took for my nerves to contract my muscles. I was wheeled back to my room to wait for the doctors to review the test. Waiting always seems longer than it really is when one is in the hospital. About an hour later, the neurological specialist arrived to talk to me about the diagnosis. The neurologist sat down and told me that I had Guillain-Barre Syndrome. I asked what that was. He explained to me that the syndrome attacks the muscles and eats away the myelin sheath (the coating around the nerves), and eventually, if not stopped, it eats into the nerves. That was the reason that I could not move or feel the sensations in my feet, legs, and hands. If this syndrome is not dealt with quickly it will, in effect, and shut down all organs and I could die. Stunned, I asked the neurologist to print out some information about this syndrome, so that I could read about it, and give this information to Judy, so that she could send it to my parents back in Elmira, NY.

Learning About Guillain-Barre Syndrome

This syndrome attacks muscles and the myelin sheath coating that protects the nerves. The diagram below shows the difference between a normal nerve, and a nerve with GBS/CIDP.

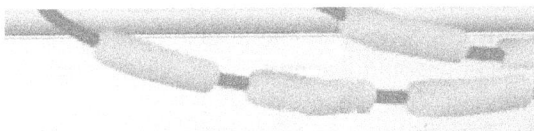

A normal nerve with its protective coating myelin sheath

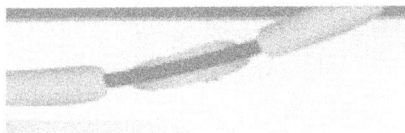

A nerve that has been attacked by GBS / CIDP

By asking me the same questions as the day before, the neurologist was able to determine just how slow or fast it was spreading throughout my body, and what treatment was best. These questions consisted of my health and wellness, if I had been, or was, sick, or if I had recently had the flu or any infections. He also wanted to know if I had any flu shots or vaccinations prior to the onset of symptoms. I responded that as far as I knew, I was healthy, I had no infections that I knew about, and that I was in good shape and participated in physical activities with my 12-year-old son.

The neurologist talked to me about how important this information was to my current status. He also explained that Guillain Barre Syndrome could shut down all of my organs, if it advanced beyond my waist. If it advanced to the upper part of my body (it was at my shoulders and it was very near my neck), next, it would effect my breathing, heart, and finally, my brain. I was becoming very scared, and in a state of mind where I did not want to accept what I was hearing from the Doctor. It was as if I was on the outside of my body, but watching my despair.

The neurologist explained to me that there are two types of treatments for GBS. One is called Plasmapheresis, and the second is High-dose immunoglobulin therapy (IVIG). He further told me that this treatment must be administered now without delay, so I agreed to this method to try to stop the progress of this syndrome, and at this time, the only one that the hospital would approve at that time was the Plasmapheresis Treatment.

At this point, he asked if I had medical insurance, and I replied that I did not. He said that he would send in a social worker, so that I could start the paper work, because these treatments are not cheap.

June 30, 2006

I was scheduled for the Plasmapheresis treatment the next day. Each treatment was to last about five hours, and there would be five treatments every other day over a period of ten days.

By now, it was becoming harder and harder to be comfortable, and the only thing that I really could do was just lay in bed with the head of the bed raised, but not too much, otherwise it would bother my waist. If I sat, I could only sit for about fifteen minutes, and no more than twenty, before it would really bother me.

The CNA that was assigned to me came in to give me the information on GBS that I had asked for so that I could read about it. After reading, I called Judy at work to tell her what was happening. That way she could look it up on the computer at her work to read what I was reading and to print up other information to send to my parents, to call them and to tell them that I was in the hospital.

Judy said that she had told Jonathan that they would both come to the hospital after work. We spent thirty minutes on the phone, and Judy told me that she would call my parents. I had spoken with my Mother a week prior, and told her what was happening to me.

My Mother called to see how I was and I told her how much worse this had become since the last time that we had talked. While on the phone, one of my doctors arrived, and he spoke to my Mother about the syndrome, and what they were doing to prevent it from progressing any further. After explaining, the Doctor handed the phone back to me. My Mother said that Judy was mailing out some information to them. More tests were needed so, I said I love you to my Mom, who said the same back to me. She would call back later.

NOTE: The information from the web that the CNA had brought to me follows. I tried to read it, but my eye-sight was a little blurry, because the GBS had also affected my eyes.

Chapter
5

What is Guillain-Barré Syndrome?

GBS

Science for the Brain, the nations leading supporter of biomedical research on disorders of the brain and nervous system more about Guillain-Barre Syndrome Studies with patients Research Literature Press Releases. NINDS is part of the National Institutes of Health.

Guillain-Barré (ghee-yan bah-ray) Syndrome is a disorder in which the body's immune system attacks part of the peripheral nervous system. The first symptoms of this disorder include varying degrees of weakness or tingling sensations in the legs. In many instances, the weakness and abnormal sensations spread to the arms and upper body. These symptoms can increase in intensity until the muscles cannot be used at all, and the patient is almost totally paralyzed. In these cases, the disorder is life threatening and is considered a medical emergency.

The patient is often put on a respirator to assist with breathing. Most patients, however, recover from even the most severe cases of Guillain-Barré syndrome, although some continue to have some degree of weakness. Guillain-Barré syndrome is rare. Guillain-Barré usually occurs a few days or weeks after the patient has had symptoms of a respiratory or gastrointestinal viral infection.

Occasionally, surgery or vaccinations will trigger the syndrome. The disorder can develop over the course of hours or days, or it may take up to 3 to 4 weeks. No one yet knows why Guillain-Barré strikes some people and not others or what sets the disease in motion. What scientists do know is that the body's immune system begins to attack the body itself, causing what is known as an autoimmune disease. Guillain-Barré is called a syndrome rather than a disease, because it is not clear that a specific disease-causing agent is involved. Reflexes such as knee jerks are usually lost. Because the signals traveling along the nerve are Slower, a nerve conduction velocity (NCV) test can give doctor clues to aid the diagnosis.

The cerebrospinal fluid that bathes the spinal cord and brain contains more protein than usual, so a physician may decide to perform a spinal tap.

Are There any Treatments?

There is no known cure for Guillain-Barre syndrome, but therapies can lessen the severity of the illness and accelerate the recovery in most patients. There are also a number of ways to treat the complications of the disease. Currently, Plasmapheresis and high-dose immunoglobulin therapy are used.

Plasmapheresis seems to reduce the severity and duration of the Guillain-Barré episode. In high-dose immunoglobulin therapy, doctors give intravenous injections of the proteins, that in small quantities, the immune system uses naturally to attack invading organism. Investigators have found that giving high doses of this immunoglobulin, derived from a pool of thousands of normal donors, to Guillain-Barré patients can lessen the immune attack on the nervous system. The most critical part of the treatment for this syndrome consists of keeping the patient's body functioning during recovery of the nervous system.

This can sometimes require placing the patient on a respirator a heart monitor or other machines that assist body function.

What is the Prognosis?

Guillain-Barré syndrome can be a devastating disorder because of its sudden and unexpected onset. Most people reach the stage of greatest weakness within the first 2 weeks after symptoms appear, and by the third week of the illness 90 percent of all patients are at their weakest. The recovery period may be as little as a few weeks or as long as a few years. About 30 percent of those with Guillain-Barré still have a residual weakness after 3 years. About 3 percent may suffer a relapse of muscle weakness and tingling sensations many years after the initial attack.

What Research is Being Done?

Scientists are concentrating on finding new treatments and refining existing ones. Scientists are also looking at the workings of the immune system to find which cells are responsible for beginning and carrying out the attack on the nervous system. The fact that so many cases of Guillain-Barré begin after a viral or bacterial infection suggests that certain characteristics of some viruses and bacteria may activate the immune system inappropriately. Investigators are searching for those characteristics. Neurological scientists, immunologists, virologists, and pharmacologists are all working collaboratively to learn how to prevent this disorder and to make better therapies available when it strikes.

What is The Myelin Sheath?

The Myelin is the insulating sheath surrounding the nerves. The white matter coating covers the nerves, enabling them to conduct impulses between the brain and other parts of the body. It consists of a layer of proteins packed between two layers of lipids.

Myelin is produced by specialized cell: oligodendrocytes in the central nervous system, and Schwann cells in the peripheral nervous system. Myelin sheaths wrap themselves around axons, the threadlike extensions of neurons that make up nerve fibers. Each oligodendrocyte can myelinate several axons.

Myelin can be destroyed by hereditary neuro-degenerative disorders such as the leukodystrophies, and by acquired diseases such as <u>multiple sclerosis</u>.

Demyelinating diseases affect more than two million people worldwide.

Other Demyelinating Diseases in Brief:

Demyelinating diseases are those in which myelin is the primary target. They fall into two main groups: acquired diseases (i.e., multiple sclerosis) and hereditary neurodegenerative disorders (i.e., the leukodystrophies). Although their causes and etiologies are different, they have the same outcome: CNS demyelination. Without myelin, nerve impulses are slowed or stopped, leading to a constellation of neurological symptoms.

Acquired Diseases

The most common of these is multiple sclerosis (MS), which usually manifests itself between a person's age of 20 and 50 years. Current estimates are that approximately 2.5 million people worldwide have MS, with between 250,000 and 350,000 cases in the United States, 50,000 cases in Canada, 130,000 cases in Germany, 85,000 cases in the United Kingdom, 75,000 cases in France, 50,000 cases in Italy, and 11,000 cases in Switzerland.

MS attacks the white matter of the central nervous system (CNS). In its classic manifestation (90% of all cases), it is characterized by alternating relapsing / remitting phases with periods of remission growing shorter over time. Its symptoms include any combination of spastic paraparesis, unsteady gait, diplopia, and incontinence.

A number of government agencies and private foundations currently support research on various myelin diseases. Some efforts focus on identifying the cause of individual diseases; others are directed toward developing therapies for arresting disease progress or preventing onset.

In contrast, little attention is being given to the problems of repairing damage already done by the disease and of restoring lost function. Laboratories working on remyelination are relatively few in number and their programs are under-funded. In addition, rivalry among researchers is intense. Laboratories tend to work in isolation, learning of each other's progress through medical journal articles, which are usually, published a year or two after experiments are completed. This fragmented approach is clearly unsuitable to regenerating CNS myelin, a complex task that requires multi-disciplinary skills.

The Scope

From myelin loss, leads to the reduction or blockage of nerve impulse conduction, myelin re-growth would logically restore conduction in diseases for which therapies capable of halting demyelination have already been found (e.g., phenylketonuria, Refsum's disease, which are treatable, mainly through restricted diets). But, regenerating myelin may also be beneficial in demyelinating diseases for which no effective treatment has been developed (e.g., multiple sclerosis). Indeed, the new myelin may well be able to withstand attack by the primary demyelinating agent, either permanently or for a long period of time. ~

June 30, 2006

I was taken to the surgical room to have a heart catheter placed in my neck for the Plasmapheresis treatment. I remained awake during the thirty minute procedure, and the catheter would remain, until all five treatments were completed. After the surgery, I was taken back to my room. Around noon, the doctor came into my room to explain about the treatment. He said that Plasmapheresis is done with a machine, and it takes about five-hour treatment. My blood would enter the machine and the blood would then be separated. My plasma and white blood cells would be removed from my blood and replaced by donated plasma would then be added to my blood and then returned back into my body. The intention was to remove the plasma and large amounts of white blood cells that were attacking my body. By doing this, we hoped that with the new, donated plasma my body would recreate new white blood cells to reverse the immune system back to normal. The first procedure would be at 4:00 pm.

Once the doctor finished explaining to me the procedure, he left. The nurse came into my room to tell me that Judy had called while I was in surgery. I returned the call to Judy to tell her what was happening, and she told me that she and Jonathan would be there, when I started this treatment.

It was very difficult for all three of us. Judy and I decided to make the situation less traumatic for Jonathan, making it easier for Jonathan by referring to Star Trek Next Generation as Captain Picard when he was placed into the Borg Consciousness. It was hard on me, but I could only imagine how hard it was for Jonathan, at his age, to watch me suffering like this.

At 4 p.m., they moved me to an ICU room for the treatment, since they did not know how I would react. I would be there for a day if everything went all right. After I arrived, I called Judy to tell her that they had moved me into an ICU room, and that it was alright for Jonathan to visit me. Then, I ordered my dinner and finished it before Judy and Jonathan arrived.

The technician arrived in my room at 5:30 pm. He began preparing the machine for the Plasmapheresis treatment, and attached the tubes to the catheter that was in my neck. My blood was filtered through this catheter into the machine separating the blood into its single parts by removing the plasma from my blood. Then the donated blood product blood was returned to my body.

Judy and Jonathan arrived at the hospital about 6:30, an hour after the treatment began. I asked Jonathan to come over and to give me a hug. I needed to let him know that I was OK. Judy told to Jonathan about the Star Trek Next Generation comparison, and Jonathan smiled and laughed. Judy asked the technician who was operating the machine about the process of Plasmapheresis treatment. The technician explained the process as Jonathan and I watched TV.

I also explained what was happening, and what they planned to do to stop the progression of the syndrome. An hour later, one of my doctors arrived in the room, and I introduced Judy and Jonathan. He was one of the five doctors that were overseeing my condition and treatment. The doctor explained the treatment, and tried to help Jonathan to understand. He told Jonathan that they were doing everything that they could do to help me to get better. Judy noticed that I was beginning to look yellow as this treatment was going on. The doctor explained that with this first treatment was the very reason why I was in ICU, because they did not know how my body would react to the treatment. He told us all that the yellowing of the skin is somewhat normal since my own blood was being removed, going into the machine, being separated, plasma was being removed, and finally, was replaced with new donated plasma. He explained that my blood was mixed back together with the new plasma, then pumped back into my body and that this treatment would continue for about five hours. They hoped to remove all of the affected white blood cells, so that my I could recreate new cells to combat and reverse my immune system. The doctor then left to continue on rounds.

After almost a hour and a half went by, before Judy and Jonathan said goodbye. They did not eat before they came over to the hospital. I said I love you to Jonathan and Judy.

Jonathan answered with, "I love you too, Daddy."

That first Plasmapheresis treatment was very hard on me, and I felt weaker during the treatment. At the same time, I was able to feel a little different feeling in my toes. I did mention this to the technician, and he was surprised to hear that.

"People usually do not feel a difference until about the third treatment" he replied.

I finally finished my first treatment, and the technician unhooked me from the machine. I rested by watching TV with the CNA continually monitoring. I was to remain in the ICU for the night and part of the next day to see how I reacted to the treatment. If I did well, I would then be taken back to a regular room.

All I could think about was Jonathan and getting better, so that I could be with him and do the things that we had once done. All I was hoping for was that the treatment would work.

Chapter
6

The First Attempt Fails

July 1, 2006

One of my physical therapists arrived around noon, and asked me to try to walk with the use of a walker. I only had about 30% of the use of my hands and arms, with weakness from my hands up my arms to the middle of my neck. Walking was difficult with the walker. The only way I could use it was to shuffle my feet along, locking my arms on the handles, while holding my whole body weight with my arms that were so weak, if my elbows collapsed, I would fall and not be able to get up on my own. Picking me up would require at least 2 CNA's. I only made it about ten feet, then I had to return to my bed to sit down, because I was so tired. My balance was terrible, and my feet felt as if I was walking on a half-filled air mattress with my eyes closed. I was experiencing partial paralysis from my waist to my toes, and unable to feel my feet shuffling along the floor. At times, I was only able to walk about twenty feet with the use of the walker. I was very frustrated, and physical therapists who came in twice a day, just do not take "no" for an answer. I knew I had to try, but it is very frustrating not to be able to do the basic things for oneself, such as walking and picking up silverware or glasses.

The first five treatments result in no problems, so I was taken to a regular room. I notified both Judy and Jonathan that I was doing ok from the treatment so far. Judy, in turn, told my parents. Now, it just remained to see how I responded from the other four treatments.

July 2, 2006

Judy and Jonathan showed up to visit, and I had my next treatment. Judy was emotionally distant from me, because her brother, Glenn was becoming worse from prostate cancer that he had been fighting for the three years. He was not expected to live past February of 2007. Both my situation and Glenn's was too much for Judy to experience at the same time.

I was still trying to make Jonathan comfortable, but I could tell that he was afraid of the whole process. Even with my assurance that they were doing everything they could, he was still scared.

With the technician monitoring the machine for my Plasmapheresis treatment, Judy and Jonathan stayed with me for two hours, and we watched our favorite TV shows, Stargate–SG1 and Stargate Atlantis. The treatment was still on-going by the time they left, and I still had about another 2 and a half hours ahead of me.

The Recovery Begins

After the next ten-days of Plasmapheresis, I was able to feel my toes a little bit, but the tingling, numbing, and swelling in my legs and hands was still present, and I could not move them. I had no muscle control in my legs to stand. I was able to move my toes a little, but it was extremely limited. I also had to use both hands to hold on to an 8 oz. or 12 oz. glass, and still needed help to sit up in the bed, since I could not do it on my won. Even though I used a walker to go from the bed to the bathroom and shower, I always needed two CNA's from the first day I was admitted. Walking was still difficult with the walker. In essence, I was not able to do anything on my own. I was having a really hard time accepting this, as I had no control over the muscles in my hand or wrist. As for the showering, it took 1 - 2 CNA's washing me and most of that time, they were ladies and I loved that part! What guy wouldn't?

From July 8th thru the 14th everything seemed to be going fine with the Plasmapheresis treatment.

Plasmapheresis **Failed**

My first treatments failed, and became even worse, and now, I could not even stand. My arms could no longer keep me upright on the walker. What little muscle control I did have previously, I no longer had. I could not even sit on the side of the bed. The partial paralysis progressed feet to my waist, into my intestines, and then, spread into my upper neck to the base of my skull. I will admit that I was terrified, now. And, watching Jonathan's terror, it was easy to see if he was wondering whether I would get better so we could do things together, again. A parent's worst nightmare is watching the scared eyes of your child. But Judy and I tried to reassure him, that I would be getting better from these treatments. While they were both there, doctors would come into my room, and try to comfort Jonathan as well. It helped Jonathan a bit, knowing that the doctors were trying to make me better.

The neurologist had been monitoring me thru all of the treatments. I had been letting him know how I had been feeling and how the treatment was working. For the past week, the therapist had been sending reports to him as well. I tried to hide my feelings, but anyone could see it in my face and feel it in my emotions. I was thinking: "What in hell was going to happen to me? Will I get better? Will I Recover anything? Will I just keep getting worst from this syndrome? I was terrified, but I tried my best not to let Jonathan know. There were times when I was feeling like just giving up, and that there was no way to beat this disease attacking me.

July 19, 2006

By now, swallowing was becoming hard, and my speech was starting to slur a little when I spoke too fast. Everything was much worse as the syndrome moved up my arms to my shoulders and neck. I was switched to a softer food diet and food cut into smaller pieces. Strangely, though, my appetite was good, and I was eating three big meals a day, except on days when I had my treatments. On those days, I only had breakfast and supper on the days. Eating softer food only lasted for a week, and then, I was back on my regular diet with no limit on the food type that I could eat.

I told the neurologist that over the past 4 days, everything had become worse and harder to do, and I was not able to move my legs at all. Another CT scan, MRI scan, and NCV were ordered for nerve conduction. The NCV showed that the syndrome had regressed and worsened to bring on the paralysis of my legs. I suggested that we do another Plasmapheresis treatment, since the first set of five worked but did not hold. The neurologist agreed, and ordered the second treatment, but this time, the plasma he ordered would not have any blood product, and would only contain plasma. By doing this, my body would have to recreate its new anti-bodies and a new immune system.

The second NCV test revealed that there was more damage to the nerves and the doctors concluded that I had GBS / Acute Relapsing CIDP. CIDP is the same as GBS, but CIDP is a more severe condition than GBS. Now, I was facing an even worse condition than the doctors had originally thought.

NOTE:
More about the GBS / CIDP and the Foundation

The Gullain-Barré Syndrome / Chronic Inflammatory Demyelinating Polyneuropathy Foundation International, a non-profit 501(c)(3) organization, was founded by Robert and Estelle
Benson as a means of helping others deal with this frightening disorder. Since its inception in 1980, self-funded with less than a handful of volunteers, this grass roots effort has become an international organization with 23,000 members in 160 chapters on five continents.

As the GBS community expanded, the Foundation chapters in the United Kingdom, Australia, India and Canada became full-fledged organizations in their own right. Since that time, the Foundation has expanded its interests and established additional groups for GBS variants, including CIDP, Children with GBS, Axonal GBS'ers, Camploybacter Precipitated GBS, and Teenagers with GBS.

Providing support and assistance to GBS/CIDP patients and their families and committed to increasing knowledge and awareness in both the public and professional communities, the Foundation provides print information and educational opportunities, sponsors worldwide meetings, lectures and support groups, hosts the bi-annual GBS/CIDP International Symposium and encourages new findings by awarding research grants for further study and experimentation.

The organization continually raises awareness by exhibiting at neurological conferences all over the world, by direct mail, by personal contact with hospitals, emergency rooms and physicians, and through their quarterly newsletter, The Communicator.

As new information becomes available, it is distributed to chapters and support groups who host local and regional meetings all over the world.

The Foundation's Medical Advisory Board includes experts in the diagnosis, treatment and research of GBS/CIDP, many of whom have authored textbooks on the disorder, and is considered to be the "think-tank" of GBS.

In keeping with its goals of education, support and research, the Foundation has extended its reach to the Internet, establishing interactive chat and discussion areas for patients, family and friends to network and communicate, and made sure that continual funding is available to support them. This website, most of which is less than three years old, is visited each month by more than 20,000 people from over 30 countries.

The Foundation is funded by contributions from individuals who have been personally touched by GBS and by corporate sources. It has been acknowledged by the Voluntary Health Agency Community as being among the top in the field, and has been acclaimed as one of the few organizations where 100% of donations are used for the purpose for which they are collected.

GBS is a worldwide disorder. There is a need for better education of the medical and lay communities about this disorder, as well as better treatments.

Additionally, because of its probable auto-immune nature, increased knowledge of GBS may well lead to a better understanding of, and treatments for, other auto-immune disorders.

Overview

What is Guillain-Barré Syndrome (GBS)?

Guillain-Barré (Ghee-yan Bah-ray) Syndrome, also called acute inflammatory demyelinating polyneuropathy and Landry's ascending paralysis, is an inflammatory disorder of the peripheral nerves – those outside the brain and spinal cord. It is characterized by the rapid onset of weakness and, often, paralysis of the legs, arms, breathing muscles and face. GBS is the most common cause of rapidly acquired paralysis in the United States today, affecting one to two people in every 100,000.

The disorder came to public attention briefly when it struck a number of people who received the 1976 Swine Flu vaccine. It continues to claim thousands of new victims each year, striking any person, at any age, regardless of gender or ethnic background.

It typically begins with weakness and/or abnormal sensations of the legs and arms. It can also affect muscles of the chest, face and eyes. Although many cases are mild, some patients are virtually paralyzed. Breathing muscles may be so weakened that a machine is required to keep the patient alive. Many patients require an intensive care unit during the early course of their illness, especially if support of breathing with a machine is required. Although most people recover, the length of the illness is unpredictable and often months of hospital care are required. The majority of patients eventually return to a normal or near normal lifestyle, but many endure a protracted recovery and some remain wheelchair-bound indefinitely.

The cause of GBS is not known and there is no effective treatment.

How is GBS Diagnosed?

Quite often, the patient's symptoms and physical exam are sufficient to indicate the diagnosis. The rapid onset of (ascending) weakness, frequently accompanied by abnormal sensations that affect both sides of the body similarly, is a common presenting picture. Losses of reflexes, such as the knee jerk, are usually found. To confirm the diagnosis, a lumbar puncture to find elevated fluid protein and electrical test of nerve and muscle function may be performed.

How is GBS Treated?

Because progression of the disease in its early stages is unpredictable, most newly diagnosed patients are hospitalized and usually placed in an intensive care unit to monitor breathing and other body functions.

Care involves use of general supportive measures for the paralyzed patient, and methods specifically designed to speed recovery, especially for those patients with major problems, such as the inability to walk. Plasma exchange (a blood "cleansing" procedure) and high dose intravenous immune globulins are often helpful to shorten the course of GBS.

Most patients, after their early hospital stay and when medically stable, are candidates for a rehabilitation program to help learn optimal use of muscles as nerve supply returns.

What Causes GBS?

The cause is not known. Perhaps 50% of cases occur shortly after a microbial (viral or bacterial) infection such as a sore throat or diarrhea. Some theories suggest an autoimmune mechanism, in which the patient's defense system of antibodies and white blood cells are triggered into damaging the nerve covering or insulation, leading to weakness and abnormal sensation.

What is Guillain-Barré syndrome?

Guillain-Barré (ghee-yan bah-ray) syndrome is a disorder in which the body's immune system attacks part of the peripheral nervous system. The first symptoms of this disorder include varying degrees of weakness or tingling sensations in the legs. In many instances, the weakness and abnormal sensations spread to the arms and upper body. These symptoms can increase in intensity until certain muscles cannot be used at all and, when severe, the patient is almost totally paralyzed. In these cases, the disorder is life threatening - potentially interfering with breathing and, at times, with blood pressure or heart rate - and is considered a medical emergency. Such a patient is often put on a respirator to assist with breathing and is watched closely for problems such as an abnormal heartbeat, infections, blood clots, and high or low blood pressure. Most patients, however, recover from even the most severe cases of Guillain-Barré syndrome, although some continue to have a certain degree of weakness.

Guillain-Barré syndrome can affect anybody. It can strike at any age and both sexes are equally prone to the disorder. The syndrome is rare, however, afflicting only about one person in 100,000. Usually Guillain-Barré occurs a few days or weeks after the patient has had symptoms of a respiratory or gastrointestinal viral infection. Occasionally surgery or vaccinations will trigger the syndrome.

After the first clinical manifestations of the disease, the symptoms can-progress over the course of hours, days, or

35

weeks. Most people reach the stage of greatest weakness within the first 2 weeks after symptoms appear, and by the third week of the illness 90 percent of all patients are at their weakest.

What causes Guillain-Barré syndrome?

No one yet knows why Guillain-Barre-- which is not contagious—strikes some people and not others. Nor does anyone know exactly what sets the disease in motion.

What scientists do know is that the body's immune system begins to attack the body itself, causing what is known as an autoimmune disease. Usually the cells of the immune system attack only foreign material and invading organisms.

In Guillain-Barré syndrome, however, the immune system starts to destroy the myelin sheath that surrounds the axons of many peripheral nerves, or even the axons themselves (axons are long, thin extensions of the nerve cells; they carry nerve signals). The myelin sheath surrounding the axon speeds up the transmission of nerve signals and allows the transmission of signals over long distances.

In diseases in which the peripheral nerves' myelin sheaths are injured or degraded, the nerves cannot transmit signals efficiently. That is why the muscles begin to lose their ability to respond to the brain's commands, commands that must be carried through the nerve network. The brain also receives fewer sensory signals from the rest of the body, resulting in an inability to feel textures, heat, pain, and other sensations. Alternately, the brain may receive inappropriate signals that result in tingling, "crawling-skin," or painful sensations. Because the signals to and from the arms and legs must travel the longest distances, they are most vulnerable to interruption. Therefore, muscle weakness and tingling sensations usually first appear in the hands and feet and progress upwards.

When Guillain-Barré is preceded by a viral or bacterial infection, it is possible that the virus has changed the nature of cells in the nervous system so that the immune system treats them as foreign cells. It is also possible that the virus "makes the immune system itself less discriminating about what cells it recognizes as its own, allowing some of the immune cells, such as certain kinds of lymphocytes and macrophages, to attack the myelin. Sensitized T -lymphocytes cooperates with B - lymphocytes to produce antibodies against components of the myelin sheath and may contribute to destruction of the myelin. Scientists are investigating these and other possibilities to find why the immune system goes awry in Guillain-Barré syndrome and other autoimmune diseases. The cause and course of Guillain-Barré syndrome is an active area of neurological investigation, incorporating the cooperative efforts of neurological scientists, immunologists, and virologists.

How is Guillain-Barré Syndrome Diagnosed?

Guillain-Barré is called a syndrome rather than a disease because it is not clear that a specific disease-causing agent is involved. A syndrome is a medical condition characterized by a collection of symptoms (what the patient feels) and signs (what a doctor can observe or measure). The signs and symptoms of the syndrome can be quite varied, so doctors may, on rare occasions, find it difficult to diagnose Guillain-Barré in its earliest stages.

Several disorders have symptoms similar to those found in Guillain-Barre, so doctors examine and question patients carefully before making a diagnosis. Collectively, the signs and symptoms form a certain pattern that helps doctors differentiate Guillain-Barré from other disorders. For example, physicians will note whether the symptoms appear on both sides of the body (most common in Guillain-Barré) and the quickness with which the symptoms appear (in other disorders, muscle weakness may progress over months rather than days or weeks). In Guillain-Barré, reflexes such as knee jerks are usually lost. Because the signals traveling along the nerve are slower, a nerve conduction velocity (NCV) test can give doctor clues to aid the diagnosis In Guillain-Barré patients, the cerebrospinal fluid that bathes the spinal cord and brain contains more protein than usual. Therefore, a physician may decide to perform a spinal tap, a procedure in which the doctor inserts a needle into the patient's lower back to draw cerebrospinal fluid from the spinal column.

How is Guillain-Barré treated?

There is no known cure for Guillain-Barré syndrome. However, there are therapies that lessen the severity of the illness and accelerate the recovery in most patients. There are also a number of ways to treat the complications of the disease.

Currently, plasma exchange (sometimes called Plasmapheresis) and high-dose immunoglobulin therapy are used. Both of them are equally effective, but immunoglobulin is easier to administer. Plasma exchange is a method by which whole blood is removed from the body and processed so that the red and white blood cells are separated from the plasma, or liquid portion of the blood. The blood cells are then returned to the patient without the plasma, which the body quickly replaces. Scientists still don't know exactly why plasma exchange works, but the technique seems to reduce the severity and duration of the Guillain-Barré episode. This may be because the plasma portion of the blood contains elements of the immune system that may be toxic to the myelin.

In high-dose immunoglobulin therapy, doctors give intravenous injections of the proteins that, in small quantities, the immune system uses naturally to attack invading organisms. Investigators have found that giving high doses of this immunoglobulin, derived from a pool of thousands of normal donors, to Guillain-Barré patients can lessen the immune attack on the nervous system. Investigators do not know why or how this works, although several hypotheses have been proposed.

The use of steroid hormones has also been tried as a way to reduce the severity of Guillain-Barré, but controlled clinical trials have demonstrated that this treatment not only is not effective but also may even have a deleterious effect on the disease.

The most critical part of the treatment for this syndrome consists of keeping the patient's body functioning during recovery of the nervous system. This can sometimes require placing the patient on a respirator, a heart monitor, or other machines that assist body function. The need for this sophisticated machinery is one reason why Guillain-Barré syndrome patients are usually treated in hospitals, often in an intensive care ward. In the hospital, doctors can also look for and treat the many problems that can afflict any paralyzed patient - complications such as pneumonia or bedsores.

Often, even before recovery begins, caregivers may be instructed to manually move the patient's limbs to help keep the muscles flexible and strong. Later, as the patient begins to recover limb control, physical therapy begins. Carefully planned clinical trials of new and experimental therapies are the key to improving the treatment of patients with Guillain-Barré syndrome. Such clinical trials begin with the research of basic and clinical scientists who, working with 'clinicians, identify new approaches to treating patients with the disease.

What is the Long-term Outlook for Those with Guillain-Barré Syndrome?

Guillain-Barré syndrome can be a devastating disorder because of its sudden and unexpected onset. In addition, recovery is not necessarily quick. As noted above, patients usually reach the point of greatest weakness or paralysis days or weeks after the first symptoms occur. Symptoms then stabilize at this level for a period of days, weeks, or, sometimes, months. The recovery period may be as little as a few weeks or as long as a few years. About 30 percent of those with Guillain-Barré still have a residual weakness after

3 years. About 3 percent may suffer a relapse of muscle weakness and tingling sensations many years after the initial attack.

Guillain-Barré syndrome patients face not only physical difficulties, but emotionally painful periods as well. It is often extremely difficult for patients to adjust to sudden paralysis and dependence on others for help with routine daily activities. Patients sometimes need psychological counseling to help them adapt.

What Research is Being Done?

Scientists are concentrating on finding new treatments and refining existing ones. Scientists are also looking at the workings of the immune system to find which cells are responsible for beginning and carrying out the attack on the nervous system. The fact that so many cases of Guillain-Barré begin after a viral or bacterial infection suggests that certain characteristics of some viruses and bacteria may activate the immune system inappropriately. Investigators are searching for those characteristics. Certain proteins or peptides in viruses and bacterial maybe the same, as those found in myelin, and the generation of antibodies to neutralize the invading viruses or bacteria could trigger the attack on the myelin sheath. As noted previously, neurological scientists, immunologists, virologists, and pharmacologists are all working collaboratively to learn how to prevent this disorder and to make better therapies available when it strikes.

Where can one get More Information?

For more information on neurological disorders or research programs funded by the National Institute of Neurological Disorders and Stroke, contact the Institute's Brain Resources and Information Network (BRAIN) at:

BRAIN
P.O. Box 5801
Bethesda, MD 20824
(800) 352-9424
www.ninds.nih.gov

GBS/CIDP Foundation International
P.O. Box 262
Wynnewood, PA 19096
info@gbsfi.com
www.gbsfi.com
tel. 610-667-0131

Chapter
7

Acute Relapsing CIDP, or...

Chronic Inflammatory Demyelinating Polyneuropathy (CIDP)

July 14, 2006

I was diagnosed with Chronic Inflammatory Demyelinating Polyneuropathy (CIDP), a neurological disorder characterized by progressive weakness and impaired sensory function in the legs and arms. The disorder, which is sometimes called Chronic Relapsing Polyneuropathy, is caused by damage to the myelin sheath (the fatty covering that wraps around and protects nerve fibers) of the peripheral nerves. Although it can occur at any age, and in both genders, CIDP is more common in young adults, and in men more so than women. It often appears with symptoms that include tingling or numbness (beginning in the toes and fingers), progressing to weakness in the arms and legs, loss of deep tendon reflexes (areflexia), fatigue, and abnormal sensations. CIDP is closely related to Guillain-Barre syndrome and it is considered the chronic counterpart of that acute disease. Below are several descriptions of this disease and its treatment.

Treatment

Treatment for CIDP includes corticosteroids, such as prednisone, which may be prescribed alone or in combination with immunosuppressant drugs. Plasmapheresis (plasma exchange) and intravenous immunoglobulin (IVIg) therapy are effective. IVIg may be used even as a first-line therapy.

Physiotherapy may improve muscle strength, function and mobility, and minimize the shrinkage of muscles and tendons and distortions of the joints.

Prognosis

The course of CIDP varies widely among individuals. Some may have a bout of CIDP followed by spontaneous recovery, while others may have many bouts with partial recovery in between relapses. The disease is a treatable cause of acquired neuropathy and initiation of early treatment to prevent loss of nerve axons is recommended. However, some individuals are left with some residual numbness or weakness.

Research

The NINDS supports a broad program of research on disorders of the nervous system, including CIDP. Much of this research is aimed at increasing the understanding of these disorders and finding ways to prevent, treat, and cure them.

Overview

What is (Chronic Inflammatory Demyelinating Polyneuropathy) CIDP?

CIDP (Chronic Inflammatory Demyelinating Polyneuropathy) is a rare disorder of the peripheral nerves characterized by gradually increasing weakness of the legs and, to a lesser extent, the arms. It is cause by damage to the covering of the nerves, called myelin. It can start at any age and in both genders. Weakness occurs over two or more months. Characteristics of CIDP that help support its diagnosis are described below.

How is CIDP Diagnosed?

The CIDP patient typically presents with difficulty walking, which progressively worsens over a few months. Tingling or other abnormal sensations may also be experienced if the patient's sensory nerve myelin is damaged. Physical examination will usually show loss of reflexes, such as the knee and ankle jerk. Evaluation by a neurologist will often include an electrical test, a nerve conduction velocity - electromyography study. It shows slowing of conduction of electrical signals or even blocked conduction. A spinal tap, to analyze cerebrospinal fluid, will typically show elevated protein with normal cells to help confirm the diagnosis. Patients with variants of CIDP, such as multifocal motor neuropathy, may only show slowing of conduction in some motor nerves to muscles. Your doctor may obtain blood and urine tests, including analysis of proteins, to look for causes of CIDP.

How is CIDP Treated?

Several treatment options are available. Prednisone, similar to protective anti-inflammatory corticosteroids that are normally made by the body, may be used as an initial treatment for several reasons. It often improves strength, can be conveniently taken by mouth and is inexpensive. Side effects can limit its use. Two other approaches have often been found helpful. High dose intravenous immune globulins (IVIG), protective blood proteins obtained from healthy volunteers, can be readily given through an arm vein. In another treatment, called plasma exchange (PE), or plasmapheresis, some of the patient's blood is removed and the blood cells returned without the liquid plasma portion of the patient's blood. It may work by removing harmful antibodies contained in the plasma. Treatment of CIDP is somewhat of an art. If a patient shows good improvement with an initial treatment but again evolves weakness it may be repeated or another therapy may be tried.

What Causes CIDP?

Current theory holds that the body's immune system, which normally protects it, perceives myelin as foreign and attacks it. Just what starts this process is not clear. Some patients are found to have abnormal proteins in their blood, and these may facilitate damage.

Chronic Inflammatory Demyelinating Polyneuropathy (CIDP)

Description

Chronic inflammatory demyelinating polyneuropathy (CIDP) is a neurological disorder that results in slowly progressive weakness and loss of feeling in the legs and arms. It is caused by the body's immune system inappropriately reacting against and damaging myelin. Myelin surrounds the peripheral nerves and acts like an insulator so that the nerves can conduct impulses properly. It is closely related to Guillain-Barré syndrome (GBS). However, GBS develops acutely (over hours-days) whereas CIDP usually develops slowing (over weeks-months).

CIDP can occur at any age and in both sexes, but is more common in men than women.

Symptoms include tingling, numbness or altered feeling, which often begins in the feet and hands, weakness of the arms and legs, fatigue and aching pain in the muscles.

Treatment

Treatment for CIDP is aimed at suppressing the immune system. First line treatment is usually with intravenous immunoglobulin. If this is not available, plasmapheresis (plasma exchange) or oral medications, which suppress the immune system such as steroids, may be used.

Physiotherapy may improve muscle strength, function and mobility, and minimize the development of contractures.

Prognosis

The course of CIDP varies widely among individuals. Some may have a bout of CIDP followed by spontaneous recovery, while others may have many bouts with partial recovery in between relapses. The disease is a treatable cause of acquired neuropathy and initiation of early treatment to prevent loss of nerve cells is recommended. However, some individuals are left with some residual numbness or weakness.

Mayo Clinic neurologists Jerry Swanson, M.D., and colleagues answer select questions from readers…

Answer

Chronic inflammatory demyelinating polyneuropathy, also called chronic relapsing polyneuropathy, occurs when the immune system mistakenly attacks peripheral nerves. This disorder occurs in different forms. The most common manifestation is slowly progressive weakness in the arms and legs.

Chronic inflammatory demyelinating polyneuropathy may follow a viral infection and can be recurrent. Signs and symptoms — which usually develop slowly over weeks and progress over several months — may include:

- Weakness in the arms, feet, legs and face
- Tingling and numbness in the arms, legs, and hands
- Muscle aches
- Fatigue

Without treatment, chronic inflammatory demyelinating polyneuropathy usually does not improve.

Treatment may include:

- Corticosteroids, such as prednisone
- Intravenous immunoglobulin (IVIG)
- Plasma exchange (Plasmapheresis)
- Physical therapy

For my CIPD, treatments continued, and my neurologist ordered a breathing test on a daily schedule, along with a blood test every three days. He also ordered heparin shots twice a day for about three weeks, since I was not able to get up and move around due to the partial paralysis from the waist to the lower extremities.

After the first two treatments of the second set of Plasmapheresis, I again felt a little relief and even was able to move my big toe a little bit. My hands and arms were still weak in strength. We knew this was should work, and it should stop the progression of this syndrome, but we proceeded with caution, hoping that the syndrome relapse would reverse as well. But, the treatment did not work, and the doctors told me that from my neck, it would progress to my upper organs, into my neck, and finally, my brain, while from my waist, it would move into my lower organs, and they would start begin to fail.

August 1, 2006

The social worker at the hospital, came into my room to talk to me about the arrangements that were being made to send me to Franklin Park Assistant Living Care Center.

August 6, 2006

After the second set of five treatments of the plasmapheresis and the next five days, things were looking favorable for me. There were no signs of relapsing at this point.

I asked Judy if I could move in with them for a while, instead of going to the assisted living, but Judy refused. The social worker had one of the personal workers from Franklin Park Living Care Center come over to meet with me and to tell me about Franklin Park. The following day, Felecia came over to meet with me to tell me about the roommate that I would be sharing the room with whose name was Gorge. She also talked about the nurses and the CNA'S that would be taking care of me, and told me that they were expecting my arrival, as well as the therapists, who would be assigned to my therapy treatments. Felecia also told me about the facility and the other workers. Felecia said that when my doctor felt that I could be released from the hospital, I would be taken to Franklin Park Assistant Living Care Center.

August 14, 2006

My neurologist finally told me that he was signing the release papers, so that I could be sent to Franklin Park Assistant Living Center. He wished me well on my recovery, and said that he would still remain my neurologist, after I left the hospital, and I would have follow up visits with him on a regular basis.

From June 28 through July 10, Judy brought Jonathan to see me three times a week, then the following two weeks, I only saw Jonathan twice a week, then once a week. The last two weeks, when I was still in the hospital, Judy did not bring Jonathan to visit me at all.

Two days before I was moved to the nursing home, I called Judy to tell her, and she let me talk to Jonathan for a little bit. My mother also called me, and I gave my mom the name, address, and phone number of the nursing home.

Chapter
8

Franklin Park Assistant Living Center

August 15, 2006

At eight a.m., I woke and ordered my breakfast. Two CNA's collected my belongings and placed them in two bags at eleven o'clock. They helped me dress, and I was ready to go to the assisted living center, since I had no place to go to live. A wheelchair would be my only way to move for 100 % of the time.

My thoughts started to drift, as I began to take in the events of the past three months and even more about the CIDP syndrome. I also knew I had to accept the fact that I would be in a wheelchair and only be able to walk about ten to forty feet with the use of the walker and I would need assistance from an aid who would have to be at my side at all times. Even though I knew that my immune system had been reversed to its normal state of existence, I was still worried about being sent to the home for recovery. But my neurologist, Dr. Machanic, M.D., who had been my neurologist since day one in the emergency room, had told me that the healing process would take time. He also explained that the healing can take several years and the exact amount of time was still unknown, but the worst was over.

When transportation arrived at eleven thirty, I was lifted into the wheelchair by one of the drivers, and the lady gathered my two bags of belongings and I was wheeled out of the room, stopping long enough to pick up the transfer papers at the nurse's station. Then, down on the elevator, and out of the hospital to the van.

I arrived at Franklin Park Assistant Living Care Center just after twelve p.m. Donnel (one of my nurses) was waiting at the front desk to sign the papers, releasing me from the

Medical Transport Service. He introduced himself, and escorted me to my room, after waiting for the previous week for my arrival.

After reaching my room, Donnel introduced me to my roommate Gorge, who was from northwestern New York in the Buffalo and Oswego area. Within fifteen minutes, the administrator, the Nurse, and the CNA's checked me in and I signed after many questions about my current status. They also wanted to know what needs I had, and asked me what I could or could not do on my own.

I really didn't want to be here, but in my condition, I had no choice at all. I needed help to the bathroom, daily help dressing, showering, and shaving, along with daily therapy.

After all the paperwork was completed, I settled in and called Judy and Jonathan to give them my room and phone number as well as the floor, however there was no phone in the room unless I paid for one. That evening my mother called me, and after we talked for a little bit, I also talked to my dad.

Over the next few days, the nurses and CNA's on the first and second floors became familiar with me. But, still, I kept to myself for a while, since I was still trying to cope with the syndrome and being in a wheelchair. I had a very hard time accepting my situation and my surroundings.

By the time two weeks rolled by, I started to relax, but still kept to myself. A couple of the CNA's on my floor introduced me to couple of the other CNA's, and some residents on my floor and the second floor. They helped me by asking me about my work, and I told them about having worked in retail and as a security officer. I also told them about my book publishing company and books that I had written and published. They were very interested, and eventually, started buying my books as well as borrowing the books to read.

The nurses, CNA's, and residents suggested that I should write about my experience. I truly thought I'd consider it because those at Rose Hospital had suggested the same thing. At that time, though, I really had no desire to write about it.

At times in my life, I had thought about writing about the experience, but I really was not wanting to share it with others. However, I was writing on one of my continuing stories of Kiser, and that was all that I really wanted to think about. It kept my mind off of my situation. And, in addition, my thoughts were also on my son Jonathan from the time I woke up till the time I went to sleep.

For the first three and a half months, I spent my life in a wheelchair. I could slowly feel my strength was returning just a little. But, I was also withdrawn and depressed, and I had no desire to be around any one.

During my first day at the nursing home, I tried calling Judy, because I wanted to hear how Jonathan was doing in school. I also wanted to see Jonathan more than the once a month Judy would bring him. Being unable to leave without someone to take me outside of the center was very hard, and seeing my son would have made it so much better.

In my therapy, I had to relearn how to walk and to get my leg muscles working with the use of the walker by using parallel bars. I had to hold my bodyweight up with my arms, since my legs and waist could not do so, and I also had therapy on the two to three step stairway.

On Thanksgiving of 2006, Judy and Jonathan came to take me to Judy's home, where we had Thanksgiving together. I enjoyed every moment that I had with Jonathan, even for only an hour or two. On some Fridays if I knew Judy and Jonathan were coming over to watch Stargate with me, I would buy pizza if I had the money, and occasionally, my parents would send me money as well.

In November and December of 2006, I was able to dress on my own and to take care of some of my persona needs. But, I still needed a CNA close by for assistance in case I fell. The muscles in my legs and in my waist were still very weak, and I was still using the wheelchair, but I was trying to use the walker.

August 15th 2006 – November 2006

My recovery felt very slow to me. I was learning how to get in and out of the wheelchair, and from the bed to a regular chair. I was also standing up from the wheelchair and sitting back down to work the muscles in my arms and legs. I needed to use my arms to lift my body, since my leg muscles were not able to do that part of the work. I also had to do hands, arms, feet, and leg exercises along with working the muscles in my waist, so they could remember how they worked in the past. I was physically exhausted.

In October of 2006, I received a letter from Social Security denying my disability. I had to do an appeal for a hearing. The next letter that I received declared that the SS Office had received my appeal, and that it would take fourteen to sixteen months to receive a hearing date. This was not making things easier for me. I was receiving no money by now. I just wanted to be alone. The only time that changed was when Judy would call so that Jonathan and I could talk.

I still needed continuing help with showers and shaving. But, by the end of February and through the end of April, all I needed was to have my CNA around in case I slipped and fell during personal needs.

During the whole time at Franklin Park Assistance Living Care Center, my two therapists, Sharon and Brenda, pushed me in fighting the battle of the syndrome. They pushed my nerves to regain their connections to work my muscles the way they did prior to the illness.

I also have to thank my CNA's and a couple of the residents for pushing me to get myself up to do things, even if it was just going outside for their social gatherings, or to play a couple games of Chess with one of the workers. They also pushed me to work on writing my fifth book, "A World-Bridger from a Distant World".

When March 2007 arrived, I received a letter from Medicaid, saying they were denying me assistance as well. I now had absolutely no income, and the nursing home was asking me to leave. They were generous in giving me time to get help. So, I called my parents, telling them with Medicaid being denied, I needed to leave the nursing home by the end of April 2007.

I also asked Judy if I could live with her and Jonathan. Judy would not let me come back. I called my parents back and told my Mother what Judy said. My Mother called to talk to Judy about me staying with her and Jonathan. And, like me, Judy refused to have me stay with them.

I had no money and no place to go. After two days had passed, my Mother called me and said that they would fly me back to their home in Elmira, NY. They wanted me stay with them as I healed, and as I waited for my SS disability appeal date. I hoped that I would be approved, so that I could get back to Denver, Colorado, to be with Jonathan.

In April of 2007, my stay at the nursing home was coming to an end, so I asked Sharon to help me with walking up and down a story of steps. At first it was hard, physically exhausting, and I was only able to do it once a day every other day. On the second week, I was doing it once a day, every day. The third and fourth week saw me trying to walk up and down the steps a couple times a day. My parents had a two-story house and the bedrooms and the bathroom were on the second floor. I knew that I had to push myself so that I could walk up and down the steps at my parent's house.

Chapter
9

Medical Assistance Denied

Back in the 3rd week of June of 2006, I had applied for disability and Medicaid. That was right before I was admitted to the hospital. I again applied for Medicaid after being admitted in the hospital on June 29, 2006. I also applied for Social Security disability on July 18, 2006 by phone, while I was still in the hospital.

In September of 2006, I resubmitted the forms for Medicaid, while I was in the nursing home. The whole time that I was in the hospital and in the nursing home, all Medicaid was able to say that the Medicaid was pending. Now with SSD, all they were able to say was that SSD was pending as well.

I tried to keep all of my discouragements, mood changes, and depression to myself. Then, on October 12, 2006, I received a letter from SSD stating that SSD was denied. They did not think that I would meet their requirements of being disabled for the minimum of 1 year. So I started the process for an appeal hearing. I received a letter from SSD stating that they had received my form for an appeal and that it could take 14 to 16 months before I would receive a hearing date.

Medicaid was still pending at that time in November of 2006. In February 2007, Medicaid contacted Franklin Park Assistant Living Care Center, saying that my Medicaid had been denied. At that time Cindy, the Administrator, contacted their attorney to see what he could do to have my Medicaid approved. He was unsuccessful, and it was the end of March of 2007. I also received a letter from Medicaid, denying my Medicaid assistance. I had no money at all and no assistance in Denver, Colorado. Since everything had been denied, the nursing home told me that I would have to leave. So, I contacted my parents back in Elmira, New York to let them know what was going on. My parents also contacted my sister Tammy, who is an accountant at a nursing home and works with Medicaid assistance. She looked into the matter, but could not find anything that could help my case.

So my parents and I talked about what we could do. The first thing was to see how long Franklin Park was going to give me to leave. I asked Cindy the Manager and the social worker how much time I had, before I had to go. They said that they would give me at least a month. I mentioned that I needed until at least the end of April to figure things out. They said that would be fine and if I needed a little more time they would allow it.

My mother and I contacted Judy again to see if I could stay there with her. I had asked Judy this same question many times over the years of us being together and every time she responded with, no way, and stop asking. I still asked her about us being together and her answer was still no way, even with what I was going through with this syndrome. Even after I had come very close to maybe even dieing from this syndrome when I was in the hospital.

One of my friends Lori mentioned that she would be able to help and let me stay at her place. But she had been having a hard time herself and she really did not have room for me in her place. She was not working that much and she moved around and I needed a stable place since I could not get around on my own. So I called my parents back after a week of trying to figure things out and told them that I had no place to stay. So my parents sent money to Carolyn another one of my friends so she could buy a plane ticket so that I could head back to Elmira, New York.

The plan was for me to stay with my parents until one of two things happened. First I would stay in Elmira, until I received SSD and then I would return to Denver. The second was that if it did not become approved then I had to wait until I healed, so that I could go back to work and save money to return to Denver.

Temporarily Returning to Elmira, New York

April 15, 2007

My friend, Carolyn, received the check from my parents, and then contacted me to see which preference I had for an airline. Once I told her, she purchased my airline ticket for me, on April 29, departing at 3 p.m.

April 17, 2007

Judy took me to a store, because it was about time for Jonathan's 13th birthday. Judy agreed to let Jonathan be with me on his birthday. Then, we picked up Jonathan from school and we all went Judy's home to visit.

April 21, 2007

Carolyn took me to buy a suitcase for my trip. It was also my 41st birthday. When Carolyn arrived at the nursing home, I signed out, and she handed me the rest of the money from the check. Since Jonathan's 13th birthday was on May 4, and I would not be in Denver, we decided to celebrate our birthdays together. After I bought a few things, Carolyn picked up Judy and Jonathan, and the four of us went to a restaurant for lunch for our birthdays. I gave Jonathan the things that Judy had told me that he wanted – action figures from the movie "The Pirates of The Caribbean".

April 29, 2007

I got up at 6 am and had breakfast, but I was feeling upset and sad that I had to leave Denver and Jonathan, and not knowing when I would be able to return home to be with him again. Carolyn picked up Judy and Jonathan, then to the living center in order to pick me up to take me to the airport.

By the time I had arrived, I was ready and they loaded my things into Carolyn's van. I talked with Jonathan, and that I would be back as soon as I could, and we would be together again. I also told him that things would be all right, and I would call every couple of weeks to let him know how I was doing and, most importantly, I would be missing him all the time.

As we arrived at the airport, I asked for assistance, and we said bye to each other. I hugged Jonathan, and him, once more, that I would be thinking of him all the time. I did tell him that he needed to behave and not cause trouble while I was gone. I knew he would miss him as much as he would miss me.

Chapter
10

A Long Road Ahead

All I could think about during the long flight from Denver to Elmira was the time that I would miss seeing Jonathan doing things with him.

I arrived at 10 p.m., and my Father picked me up at the airport to head home. Dad asked if I had eaten. I hadn't, and my Dad asked if Burger King or McDonald's would be ok. I said Burger King would be fine, and stopped to buy me a late dinner.

When we pulled into the driveway of my Parent's house, Mom came out and gave me a hug. She said that she loved me, had missed me, and how glad that I was home. I told my Mom it was good to be back, but I wished it had not been in this condition. I told her that Jonathan was really all I could think about, and to be away from him was very painful. Dad carried my suitcase and briefcase inside and we followed Mom inside. I called Jonathan, and we talked for half an hour. I told Jonathan that I loved him, missed him and that I would call to talk to him every week. I knew the time apart would be time that could never be replaced.

I ate my dinner, while I spoke to Mom and Dad about the syndrome that I had, how I had almost died, and my recovery until about 1a.m. I wanted to try to regain 100% of my health, again or at least as close as possible to my life, before this syndrome attacked my body. I told them that the Plasmapheresis helped a great deal in reversing my auto immune system to normal, until we all grew tired, and decided it was time to go to bed.

April 30, 2007

My Mother called their family doctor to make an appointment for me, so that I could have access to him in order to continue recovering from the GBS/Acute Relapsing CIDP syndrome. The doctor's office at the Medical Art Building at Saint Joseph's Hospital was able to set an appointment for the end of May.

When I left the assisted living center in Denver, I had enough medication to last for about a month and a half, so I would not have to refill these immediately.

Over the next few weeks, my Parent's neighbors, who had known me since the day I was born came to visit. They were all glad that I was doing well and healing. A couple of my best friends were still living a couple of houses down from them, and it was great seeing them. Even though I talked with them about my condition with my friends. it was still hard for me to accept I had been devastated with the syndrome.

My Uncle, Mom's brother, and his family also came to visit. Even some of my Parents' friends I had known forever, visited me visited and wanted me to come over to their home to visit when my Parents came to see them. Nevertheless, there were many times, however, that I just wanted to be alone to deal with my condition.

It was the end of May, and I kept my appointment with our family doctor. He also told me to apply for Medicaid, and Mom and I went to the hospital's Medicaid office to apply. Within three days, I was approved for Medicaid assistance! If I had been approved for Medicaid when I was in the hospital for six weeks, I would never have had to leave Denver. At least I had it now, but I was still puzzled as to why I was not approved Denver, even with the neurologist's request. Our family doctor set appointments with a physical therapist for the end of June, and also with a neurologist for August, all while he monitored my condition.

Physical therapy continued in Elmira from the end of June of 2007 through February 2008. During this time, I had only healed from the middle of both lower legs to about five inches above both ankles, continuing to work its way down to my toes, and the muscles from my waist to my ankles. I was still weak, still unbalance, and still in need of the use of the cane to help me walk. Even though, I was healing from my shoulders to my wrists, the muscles in my arms continued to have muscles spasms, and my fingers would tighten from both of my arm muscles.

The normal time for nerves to heal is about 1 inch per month, if the nerves are not badly damaged, but it can take up to two to three months just to heal 1 inch. However, if the nerves are severely damaged, it can take the nerve a year, to several years to heal.

Being away from Jonathan was the hardest part of everything. Most of my time was spent outside on my Parents' front porch or on the patio. My Parents had two stray cats that had adopted them. One cat was brown and black striped and called Tiger, and no one could get near him, unless he adopted you into his family. It took Tiger about two months to finally approve me as part of his family. Until he did, however, he would follow me, when I walked up and down the block. Afterward, he would sit on my lap every time that I was outside and then he would walk beside me. Then one day during the summer told Tiger that since he was by himself and other cats were picking on him, he should find a kitty friend. Strangely enough, about two weeks later Tiger brought a friend home. This cat was twice the size of Tiger and black with yellow eyes. I, now, had two cats that would sit on my lap and sleep in my arms at the same time. Since Tiger was a small cat, I held him in my arms and the other cat (Blacky) would lay on my lap or sit on my shoulders if Tiger was on my lap. They both walked beside me all the time on our walks. It was great having these two cats around me all the time. Between the cats and talking to Jonathan, it made this much more bearable.

In the fall of 2007. the nerves that are five inches above both ankles were healing an inch every six months. This was the most damaged area, and would take the longest time to heal. The actual length of time that it would take my body to completely heal from this syndrome was totally unknown, because no two people's bodies are the same and no two people heal the same.

As of November 2007, I was having problems mentally, physically, and emotionally. I had a lot of stress, did not want to be around people at times, and preferred to be by myself. I was started to experience forearm muscles periodically tightening, and affected my fingers. They would close shut or tighten to where I needed to massage them in order to relax the muscles, which in turn, would relax the muscles in my fingers.

As December 2007 rolled around, I called Judy and Jonathan to see what Jonathan would like for Christmas. Of course his main toys that he loved were Lego's, so I bought a couple of sets for him as well as some other toys. He loved them and everything else that I bought for him and the things my Parents bought and sent.

In the middle of January 2008, what had been an acceptable sleep habit (2a.m. – 9 or 10a.m.) for me, reversed back to normal, and I was feeling alright with the amount of sleep that I was receiving. That was until around the middle of January of 2008, when I was not falling asleep until 4a.m. – 5a.m., and waking around 10:30 a.m. – 11a.m. I was staying in bed until 11:30a.m. - Noon. I was always exhausted.

July 5, 2008

Since April, the Doctor had been decreasing the Prednisone, and I was taking 17.5 mg. My feet had now healed to about 3-4 inches above both ankles, and continued down to my toes. The muscles in both of my legs had relapsed, since the healing was still working on both legs. The numbness and the weakness were still present in my ankles and I had very little muscle control. In my waist, there was still some unbalance. My hands still continued to have numbness and weakness, and at times tingling, with a lack of sensation in both hands and arms. It still affected the muscles at the base of my neck, along with my vision. When I turned my head side to side and up and down, it brought about increasing pain along with blurred vision.

In April of 2008, it began to look like this syndrome was relapsing only within the muscles, but not in the nerves, which was actually a good sign. I was paying close attention to every part of my body, the nerves and the muscles as time advanced.

In June 2008, I heard that one of my other friends from high school, Sharon, was back in Elmira. So, I got in touch with her, and she agreed to meet me. We talked about what I was going through, my son and her two boys.

In July 2008, the muscles in my forearms were still tightening and affecting my fingers. It had increased by fifty percent since January 2008. If I bent my wrist too far, it would cause the muscles in my forearms to tighten as well, and my fingers would close.

At the end of July 2008, Judy told me that she and Jonathan had been evicted, and she cut off all communication between my son and me, claiming that it was because of me they had been evicted. On top of all of that, she told our mutual friends not to tell me where they were living. Now, I had even more to worry about, and I really didn't need it. I was missing Jonathan even more than ever.

After two years and two months, I was finally approved for Social Security Disability on August 27, 2008. The SS office said that it could take another sixty – ninety days for the paper work to be completed. I was thrilled that I would be able to return to Denver, Colorado, in November of 2008. When I did return to Denver, I was determined that many things would change between Judy and me. Jonathan and I would be able to make up for this past year and a half of not being able to see each other or even talk to him on the phone.

For myself and for anyone that does come down with this type of syndrome this is not a fast recovery, but there is a recovery. This syndrome attacks the nerves and the muscles and starts at the bottom of one's body at the feet and hands, working up the body. The healing works in the opposite direction, it starts at the top and works its way down as it heals. Remember, as your body heals from top to bottom, everything below is still being attacked and it will take the body longer to heal those areas.

It was now the near the end of December of 2008, and although I had thought to return in November, I was a bit late in doing so while waiting for my SSDI, which I finally received. I was eagerly planning to return to Denver, which has been my home since May 1990. However, my Mother was concerned, that I would have a very hard time living on my own, since I had been living with my Parents since April 29, 2007. I had been dependent on them to help me to get around since it was difficult to walk, and I could not drive. I would be doing a tremendous amount of walking, once I was home, and I would be using the Denver RTD bus system to get around on my own. I told my Mother that I had been away from Jonathan far too long, and I needed to get home. I needed to find Judy and Jonathan, so that Jonathan and I could start being with each other again.

January 13, 2009

I returned to Denver, and a friend picked me up at DIA (Denver International Airport). He left me at a hotel where I stayed for a month while I called around to find a apartment.

I also started to take care of some bills from the past to look for Judy and Jonathan. I knew that Jonathan would be going to Denver South High School based on what Judy told me during the early summer of 2008. I went to the school and talked to one of the administrators. He could not give me any other information other than Jonathan was attending at the request of his Mother. The administrator did suggest that I should see a social worker, who would get in touch with the school or get a court order. So, I spent my days trying figure out how to see Jonathan and to find out where he was living. On February 11, I finally found a place. I had a friend help me move into my apartment in one day. Then, I spent the next two-three weeks unpacking, taking my time, but trying to get things done.

On March 19, I received my Colorado ID. When I was coming back on the bus at one of the bus stops by Jonathan's school, I saw Jonathan getting onto one of the buses. He had changed a lot, but as a parent you know your son. Even if you have not seen him or received any photos of him. Jonathan also recognized me. He was about two inches taller than me, and I am 6'-1½" tall, while Jonathan is about 6'-3". He was still as skinny as he was when I left a year and nine months prior. Jonathan and I talked for about twenty minutes, and I just rode the second bus to be with Jonathan and to talk and see how he was doing. I was not pleased to hear what Jonathan's Mother was doing. I was glad that Jonathan and I met on the bus that day and talked. It helped me to set my mind at ease.

My healing had begun to slow, and it was taking about one year and four months to heal one inch by now. I had healed just about four inches above both ankles as it continued to heal towards my toes. My hands were still having some nerve and muscle shaking, and the muscle tightening. It cost me a lot of money, but I was willing to do it. I needed to see him…to have our missed time together.

Chapter
11

Relapsing and a New Treatment

The syndrome had been taking a toll on all levels that is unimaginable, and only one who has been through it, or is going through it, knows the pain, depression, and frustration, and most especially – relapse.

March 26, 2009

In my case, all the activities I had been participating in caused a second relapse. I knew that it was a possibility. It triggered the nerves and the muscles in the same manner as it had back in the summer of 2006. This time, I was having a hard time walking and sitting. I was having severe pain in my hands, both feet and legs, and all the way up to my waist. I could not even sit to enjoy eating, but had to eat quickly to get back into my bed. Even personal needs became painful. After four days of intense pain, I called 911. After the hospital admitted me into a room, one of the doctors that were on call received my records. When she came into the room she told me that when she looked at my records, my name seemed familiar to her, but she could not place a face to the name. Once she saw me, she recognized me, and asked about how I had been since the last time that I had been admitted. I told her that I had been doing very well, and I had been very active, since I returned to Denver in January. I also explained that I had been doing everything on my own, and I felt that I had over compensated. But, I wanted so much to get my life back.

My doctor said that she hoped they did not have me another six weeks, and neither did I. Now that I had relapsed, I would have to begin the healing process all over again. The doctor said that they would run tests, asking if I would like to have the same neurologist that I had when this all started almost three years ago. I replied yes. It would be a great idea to have the same doctor, because he was already familiar with my case.

After my first day in the hospital and the first initial tests came back, they started to pump antibiotics into me. The doctor said that I had some type of bacteria on my feet around both ankles called Cellulitis. They continued repeat tests over the next couple of days to see if anything else had been affected. They found that my white blood cells were again working overtime, and that my white blood cell count was up twenty percent. They started a second type of antibiotics.

This time I was in the hospital from March 30 through April 9, 2009. After I finished the antibiotics, I was to make an appointment with my neurologist to start the IVIG treatment. He had already approved it while I was in the hospital, but for some reason, that appointment was not made. I kept asking the other doctors about it, and they wanted to wait until I was off the antibiotics. Of course my neurologist was not pleased to hear that, so he prescribed the treatments and had his office set up the appointment.

May 15, 2009

Three years from the first onset of GBS/Acute Relapsing CIDP, I started my first of three sets of treatments of IVIG on May 15, 2009. After the relapse, it had taken my body about two months to recover to where it had been prior to it. GBS/Acute Relapsing CIDP has a slow healing process of the nerves and of the muscles that were attacked by this syndrome. It was possible that it would take another three years to heal to arch of my feet.

August 17, 2009

My neurologist took me totally off the prednisone as of the beginning of September 2009. He continued with the

IVIG treatments for the next three years, until August of 2012.

October 30, 2009

I was still having problems with my muscles in my arms and feet. It will still take several more years to hopefully heal 100% from this syndrome. Only time will tell.

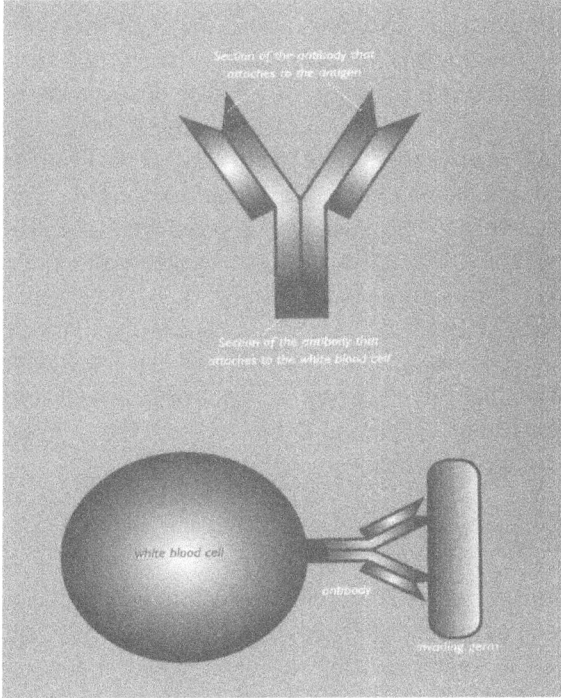

What is IVIG?

IVIG is Called - Intravenous – Immunoglobulin

An Immunoglobulin (antibody) provides the missing link between a white blood cell and the antigen on an invading germ. This connection allows the white blood cells to destroy the invaders.

1. What is it?

A blood product formed by taking antibodies from about 1,000 different donors and mixing it together. This has proven effective in several immune system disorders, including some autoimmune conditions like. CIDP.

2. How does it work?

For immune disorders where the body does not make certain antibodies, IVIG simply supplies them. For autoimmune disorder, like CIDP, the: mechanism is not as clear. It is believed that when the body's immune system is attacking itself, flooding it with antibodies from so many different people causes it to become temporarily "confused," stop the attacks, ask itself, "Wait, what am I supposed to be fighting?" and then in many instances to correctly retarget. However, this is only one theory.

Because IVIG is believed to only be effective when there is an active attack underway, it can be used with CIDP whenever there is a relapse. It is not of help with GBS after the initial attack, because it doesn't heal the myelin, it just helps reduce the attack.

3. How long does it take to have an effect?

Some patients report a combined reduction in autoimmune attack AND an anti-inflammatory effect which can lead to significant improvement within a few days. For many others, however, the benefit is in the stopping of the autoimmune attack, which keeps things from getting worse, but the healing occurs on its normal slow path.

So some will see an effect in a few days, but many will simply discover that within a month or so they are much better than they would have been if the attack had not been stopped.

In the case of GBS, studies have indicated that when given in the first few weeks, the long-term recovery period (which can be 6 months to a year) is reduced to 3 to 6 months, and the risk of permanent residual effects is often reduced. So it is not at all uncommon for people to not see any immediate effect, but still benefit significantly in the long run. The same is true with plasmapheresis, which has the same therapeutic goal: to stop the attack so the body can heal itself.

4. Why is it so expensive?

The process of collecting and mixing the antibodies from so many different people is highly complex. In addition, each individual donation must be screened for various blood-borne illnesses. In many cases, the batches are made from paid donations, which adds to the cost.

It can take over 2 months to make a single batch of IVIG. Medical insurance, including Medicaid, will normally cover IVIG for a diagnosis of CIDP at regular intervals or for GBS within the first 2 to 4 weeks.

5. Why can't we just use the much less expensive Gamma Globulin?

The regular Gamma Globulin comes from just one person. Unfortunately, it has not been shown to have the same effect as IVIG. In the case of autoimmune disorders, instead of the attack becoming "confused" and stopping, it can happen that the new antibodies simply line up with the body's original ones, making the attack even stronger. It appears to take the "flooding" effect of antibodies from many different people to stop the attack.

6. How is IVIG given?

It is an infusion, which means the liquid is slowly fed into the bloodstream through a vein. For most people, this is a "stick," like any IV. Sometimes a blood thinner is given first to keep the vein open.

The rate of infusion is a delicate balance--the faster it goes, the sooner it's over, but giving it faster can increase side effects like headaches, allergic reactions, and heart palpitations. Many nurses will experiment for the first 20 minutes or so to find a "drip rate" that seems comfortable for the patient. It is common for an adult's infusion to take 3 to 6 hours.

7. What are the most common side effects?

After the infusion, the increased level of antibodies can lead to "flu-like" symptoms, such as itchiness, low fever, and mild headaches. More specific symptoms seem to be related to allergies, but whether this is an allergy to a component of the IVIG or just the IVIG triggering an allergic reaction is not clear. These can include dryness of the mouth, rash, itchiness, and headache.

8. What can be done to reduce the side effects?

One of the most important techniques appears to be to drink plenty of fluids before and during the infusion.

However, avoid fluids with caffeine like coffee, tea, and cola. Water, juice, and Sprite seem to be helpful. Many patients report that taking Benadryl or a similar oral anti-histamine just before the infusion helps reduce rash and itching. Benadryl as an internal medication (not the skin cream) has also been reported as helpful with rashes that appear in the next day or so. Remember that whatever is going on is going on as the result of activity in the blood itself, not a contact allergy, so probably needs to be treated "from the inside out."

9. Is the treatment given at home or in the hospital?

Many doctors prefer the first treatment to be given in hospital, as a very few people (1 in 40,000) can have a very severe allergic reaction to IVIG. After the first treatment, it is often given by a home health nurse in the home. If the patient lives close to a hospital, even the first treatment may be given at home.

10. How often is the treatment given?

That varies by patient. Many CIDP patients are on a schedule of a 2, 3, or 5-day course, repeated every month to six weeks. Some people require a course of treatment only once every six months. The pattern appears to be individual. Many CIDP patients wait until they feel symptoms indicating that a new attack is underway (particularly persistent "pins and needles" in the toes or fingers lasting more than 1 day), and then call the doctor to schedule the treatment.

11. What else is in the IVIG preparation?

This depends on the brand. There will be preservatives, detergents, and possibly thinners. The exact mix and type of these will vary by brand. It can happen that a person who is allergic to the detergent or preservative in one brand will be able to use another.

12. Are there any other differences in brands?

The primary differences are in the preservatives and detergents used. There are seven different brands available in the US.

13. What is a recall and why does it happen?

Like all blood products, each lot of IVIG is tagged with a number (A lot may be 100 doses or more, depending on the method of preparation and the manufacturer.) If one of the donors to that particular lot is diagnosed with a blood-borne illness AFTER the lot was prepared, then the entire lot will have to be removed from use and destroyed. Although this is rare, it can happen. If a particular lot were, discovered to be contaminated or was improperly stored during manufacture, it may also be recalled.

14. Would recalls affect me?

Recalls normally affect only those people who STORE the products prior to their use. Most CIDP patients do not receive the IVIG until the week it will be used, so it's unlikely that recalls affect them directly. However, pharmacies, hospitals, and visiting nurse associations who administer IVIG may have to reschedule appointments if the IVIG they were intending to use is recalled and they have to wait for a new supply.

15. Where can I find out about recalls?

The National Hemophilia Foundation in the US maintains a current list of blood-product recalls on its site. This is because its members use so many different types of blood products, and generally store them in quantity. Look under medical news near the bottom of page, or in the news section. Note that most of the products shown there are not IVIG--IVIG recalls are in most years quite rare.

16. Why was there a shortage of IVIG in the US in 1997 and 1998?

There were two reasons. First, one of the major manufacturers had an equipment failure that required withdrawing a large number of lots. More significantly, however, the US Government changed its reporting procedures, requiring that anyone who had been exposed to CJD ("mad cow disease" AND a similar illness) report that as a blood-borne illness. This included people who were in the families of CJD patients, but who did not have it themselves. It also included people who had a second form, which was not likely to be blood borne. The government was reacting out of fear of a contaminated blood supply, such as had happened early on with HIV.

They set the requirements very conservatively, in advance of full scientific knowledge of how contagious CJD was. The result was that many lots had to be withdrawn, even if they contained antibodies from people who didn't have CJD themselves, but simply had a relative who did. Because the order went into effect after the IVIG had already been created, people had not necessarily been screened in advance, either. The result was that many months of production had to be recalled.

Because IVIG can take several months to make, this was an ongoing problem, and there were shortages throughout 97 and 98. In 1998, the government revised its standards as more information became known, and only actively contaminated blood had to be discarded, not the blood of relatives. In addition, better prescreening was developed. The shortage had eased by mid 1999.

IVIG is one of the blood products most vulnerable to recall when a NEW blood borne illness is discovered, because it contains antibodies from about 1,000 donors, not just one.

17. Which is better, IVIG or Plasmapheresis ("washing the blood')?

Both treatments are believed to be equally effective for CIDP and GBS. Some CIDP patients respond to one, some to the other, some to both, some to neither.

In terms of pluses and minuses, they exist on both sides. IVIG can be given at home, while plasmapheresis requires a machine that is generally available only in hospitals. IVIG requires restocking each time, while plasmapheresis uses a permanent shunt. IVIG is more expensive during shortage years otherwise costs are similar. Plasmapheresis is not affected by shortages. IVIG does not affect the levels of other medications in the blood, but plasmapheresis does, which can be tricky for patients receiving medication for thyroid or diabetes, or even antibiotics. So the decision of which to try first is an individual one.

There has been some indication that if IVIG begins to lose its effectiveness, switching to plasmapheresis for a few courses and then back to IVIG can restore the effectiveness of IVIG treatments.

18. What if both IVIG and Plasmapheresis don't work for me?

While rare, this can happen, or allergic reactions may indicate other treatments should be tried. WIG works by ADDING antibodies to the bloodstream, but because they are not coordinated in attack, they appear to confuse the body into "retargeting." Plasmapheresis works by removing the antibodies that were doing the attack, in the hopes that newly created ones will not attack the body itself. Other treatments such as immuran, azathioprine, cyclophosphamide, cyclosporin, and interferon beta are immune suppressants. These reduce the immune activity of the body. Although in some cases easier to take than the IVIG or plasmapheresis, their effect on the body is much more complex and side effects can be more severe. That is why they are second stage treatments, and need close managing.

GBS Organization of the UK
http://www.gbs.org.uk/informationJitm1

National Institute of Health report on IVIG:
http://text.nlm.nih_gpv/nih/cdc/www/8Otxt.html

GBS mailing list/support group ~ http://www.gbs.org

Red Cross page on WIG administration (for nurses)
http://www.redcross.org/plasma1pang1obu1in1aba4.htrn

Neuroland summary page on IVIG treatment (for health care professionals) http://www.neuroland.com/med/ivig.htm

National Hemophilia Foundation:
http://www.hernopia.org/

The preceding was compiled by Robin; adapted with permission from postings of the GBS et al mailing list at www.gbs.org 02/2000

This FAQ is provided for general education only--always check with your doctor for information specific to your situation, and because new knowledge and treatments are being developed all the time.

Chapter
12

Autoimmune Diseases

Autoimmunity plays a role in more than 80 diseases. Following are brief descriptions of some of the many diseases in which autoimmunity may be involved following is a list of Autoimmune Diseases. They are all caused by the immune system attacking different organs of our body. Since all these diseases have the same mechanism of action thus their treatment is essentially the same. They are treated with IVIG, steroids, plasmapheresis or other cytotoxic and immunosuppressive treatments.

List of some Auto Immune System Disorders

AUTOIMMUNE acute disseminated encephalo-myelitis (ADEM)
A flu followed by seizures and coma, causing inflammation of the brain (Encephalitis). It is an autoimmune disease.

Autoimmune Alzheimers: A memory disorder caused by autoimmune disease.

Autoimmune alopecia areata-- A disorder in which the immune system attacks the hair follicles, causing loss of hair on the scalp, face, and other parts of the body.

Autoimmune ankylosing spondylitis-- A rheumatic disease that causes inflamed joints in the spine and sacroiliac (the joints that connect the spine and the pelvis) and, in some people, inflamed eyes and heart valves.

Autoimmune aneurysms and their treatment with steroids

Autoimmune arthritis-- A general term for more than 100 different diseases that affect the joints. Many forms of arthritis and related conditions are believed to have an autoimmune component.

Autoimmune antiphospholipid Syndrome Causes Infertility recurrent abortions, stroke and thrombosis.

Autoimmune Addison's Disease The Kennedy Disease

Autoimmune Hemolytic Anemia

Autoimmune Inner Ear Disease Also known as Meniers Disease. (hearing loss, vertigo)

Autoimmune Lymphoproliferative Syndrome (ALPS)

Autoimmune Thrombocytopenic Purpura (ATP) ITP was the first disease to be approved by FDA for treatment with IVIg.

Autoimmune autism or Autistic disorder Also known as a specific entity as <u>PANDAS</u>.
(Childhood psychiatric disorders)

Autoimmune hemolytic anemia-- A condition in which immune system proteins attack the red blood cells, resulting in fewer of these oxygen-transporting cells.

Autoimmune hepatitis-- A disease in which the body's immune system attacks liver cells, causing inflammation. If not stopped, inflammation can lead to cirrhosis (scarring and hardening) of the liver and eventually liver failure.

Autoimmune Oophoritis Premature Ovarian Failure causing infertility.

Autoimmune Behcet's disease-- A condition characterized by sores in the mouth and on the genitals and by inflammation in parts of the eye. In some people, the disease also results in inflammation of the joints, digestive tract, brain, and spinal cord.

Autoimmune Bullous Pemphigoid Skin lesions

Autoimmune Cardiomyopathy A very simple treatment for end stage cardiac failure.

Autoimmune Crohn's disease-- An inflammatory disease of the small intestine or colon that causes diarrhea, cramps, and excessive weight loss.

Autoimmune Chronic Fatigue Syndrome In this condition you feel tired all the time.

Autoimmune Dermatomyositis-- A rare autoimmune disease that causes patchy red rashes around the knuckles, eyes, and other parts of the body along with chronic inflammation of the muscles. It may occur along with other autoimmune diseases such as rheumatoid arthritis or systemic lupus erythematosus.

Autoimmune Diabetes mellitus, t~De 1-- A condition in which the immune system destroys insulin-producing cells of the pancreas, making it impossible for the body to use glucose (blood sugar) for energy. Type 1 diabetes usually occurs in children and young adults.

Autoimmune Epilepsy Autoimmune In epilepsy either you pass out, forget, get angry or have uncontrolled movements of the body.

Autoimmune Kawasaki's Disease A disease affecting the skin and heart in children.

Autoimmune Glomerulonephritis-- Inflammation of the kidney's tiny filtering units, which in severe cases can lead to kidney failure.

Autoimmune Graves' disease-- An autoimmune disease of the thyroid gland that results in the overproduction of thyroid hormone. This causes such symptoms as nervousness, heat intolerance, heart palpitations, and unexplained weight loss.

Autoimmune Goodpasture's syndrome A autoimmune disease affecting the Lungs and Kidneys.

Autoimmune Guillain-Barré syndrome / CIDP--A disorder in which the body's immune system attacks part of the nervous system, leading to numb, weak limbs and, in severe cases, paralysis, treatment with IVIg, and Plasmapheresis exchange.

Autoimmune Inflammatory bowel disease-- The general name for diseases that cause inflammation in the intestine, the most common of which are ulcerative colitis and Crohn's disease.

Autoimmune Lupus nephritis-- Damaging inflammation of the kidneys that can occur in people with lupus. If not controlled, it may lead to total kidney failure.

Autoimmune Multiple sclerosis-- A disease in which the immune system attacks the protective coating called myelin around the nerves. The damage affects the brain and/or spinal cord and interferes with the nerve pathways, causing muscular weakness, loss of coordination, and visual and speech problems.

Autoimmune Myasthenia gravis-- A disease in which the immune system attacks the nerves and muscles in the neck, causing weakness and problems with seeing, chewing, and/or talking.

Autoimmune Myocarditis-- Inflamed and degenerating muscle tissue of the heart that can cause chest pain and shortness of breath. This can lead to congestive heart failure.

Autoimmune Parkinson diseases. Parkinson which causes slowness and a flexed posture with tremors is a autoimmune diseases.

Autoimmune PANDAS Pediatrics autoimmune neuropsychiatry disorders

Autoimmune Pemphigus / Demphigoid-- An autoimmune disease of the skin characterized by itching and blisters. (Excellent Article modified by cidpusa)

Autoimmune Pernicious anemia-- A deficiency of the oxygen-carrying red blood cells that often occurs in people with autoimmune diseases of the thyroid gland.

Autoimmune Polyarteritis nodosa-- An autoimmune disease that causes inflammation of the small and medium-sized arteries. This leads to problems in the muscles, joints, intestines, nerves, kidney, and skin.

Autoimmune Polymyositis-- A rare autoimmune disease characterized by inflamed and tender muscles throughout the body, particularly those of the shoulder and hip girdles.

Autoimmune Primary biliary cirrhosis-- A disease that slowly destroys the bile ducts in the liver. When the ducts are damaged, bile (a substance that helps digest fat) builds up in the liver and damages liver tissue.

Autoimmune Psoriasis-- A chronic skin disease that occurs when cells in the outer layer of the skin reproduce faster than normal and pile up on the skin's surface. This results in scaling and inflammation. An estimated 10 to 30 percent of people with psoriasis develop an associated arthritis called psoriatic arthritis.

Autoimmune Rheumatic fever-- A disease that can occur following untreated streptococcus (strep) infection. It most often affects children, causing painful, inflamed joints and, in some cases, permanent damage to heart valves.

Autoimmune Rheumatoid arthritis-- A disease in which the immune system is believed to attack the linings of the joints. This results in joint pain, stiffness, swelling, and destruction.

Autoimmune Sarcoidosis-- A disease characterized by granulomas (small growths of blood vessels, cells, and connective tissue) that can lead to problems in the skin, lungs, eyes, joints, and muscles.

Autoimmune Scleroderma-- An autoimmune disease characterized by abnormal growth of connective tissue in the skin and blood vessels. In more severe forms, connective tissue can build up in the kidneys, lungs, heart, and gastrointestinal tract, leading in some cases to organ failure.

Autoimmune siögren's syndrome-- A condition in which the immune system targets the body's moisture-producing glands, leading to dryness of the eyes, mouth, and other body tissues.

Autoimmune Systemic lupus erythematosus-- An autoimmune disease, primarily of young women, that can affect many parts of the body, including the joints, skin, kidneys, heart, lungs, blood vessels, and brain.

81

Autoimmune Thyroiditis-- An inflammation of the thyroid gland that causes the gland to become underactive. This results in symptoms such as fatigue, weakness, weight gain, cold intolerance, and muscle aches.

Autoimmune Ulcerative colitis-- A disease that causes ulcers in the top layers of the lining of the large intestine. This leads to abdominal pain and diarrhea.

Autoimmune Uveitis-- The inflammation of structures of the inner eye, including the iris (the colored tissue that holds the lens of the eye) and the choroid plexus (a network of blood vessels around the eyeball). Uveitis occurs with some rheumatic diseases, including ankylosing spondylitis and juvenile rheumatoid arthritis.

Autoimmune Vitiligo-- A disorder in which the immune system destroys pigment-making cells called melanocytes. This results in white patches of skin on different parts of the body.

Autoimmune Wegener's granulomatosis-- An autoimmune disease that damages the small and medium-sized blood vessels throughout the body, resulting in disease in the lungs, upper respiratory tract, and kidneys

Autoimmune Wilsons Disease. Liver disease with slow movements, tremor.

What are Auto Immune System Disorders?

The most common cause of all diseases in the world today is autoimmune diseases. Your own immune system acts like an invading army when it attacks you from inside. The name of the disease will depend on the location that is being attacked. The treatments for most autoimmune diseases remains about the same. Today Alzheimer's, Cancer, Heart disease, and even strokes are all caused by the immune system.

The official ranking by the N.I.H is that the *third biggest disease category* in the United States are autoimmune diseases right behind heart disease and cancer. Our clinical doctors both in the USA and Pakistan report autoimmune diseases as the number one killer and number one all over planet Earth. Since all the autoimmune diseases are mediated by the immune system the treatment for all is similar. Only one disease, Myasthenia, can be cured by Thymectomy, because the Thymus is attacking itself. Thymectomy CIDP USA has a new guide to help Myasthenia patients.

Chapter
13

Conclusion

In March 2010, the Court decided gave me the right to have Jonathan to visit me every other weekend, until Jonathan feels up to seeing me every week. This was one battle that I won so that I could have time with him. It also helped me with my emotional healing, and helped me heal much faster.

In August 2011, Jonathan decided that he would leave his Mother, to live with me full time. I told Jonathan I would welcome him, if that is what he wanted to do. And, so Jonathan moved in with me.

As 2012 rolled around, I was still healing slowly, and it was taking about 6 months for the nerves to heal, and was still about four inches above my ankles. I still had some shaking of my hands from the nerves not healing down to the wrist. However, there has not been any relapse of this syndrome since 2009.

Walking is getting easier, but I still use a cane, when I go out for anything.

When the summer of 2014, I began to think about leaving Denver, Colorado, to return to Elmira, New York. I called my Mother and explained that I was thinking about coming home. I also told her how I'd been feeling during my illness every 2 weeks, since I came back to Denver in January 2009. I also said that Jonathan and I been talking about it as well, and realized that my parents had never seen Jonathan at all! All my parents had were pictures of him. As the year went by we kept talking about leaving Colorado.

I did not know what this moving to New York would do to me, but I had the feeling I needed to leave Denver. And, that feeling escalated 2015 started. By July 2015, our decision was made. We would go home. I called my Mom and told her that Jonathan and I were going home to Elmira. We packed up our belongings, and sent fifteen boxes to my parents' home.

My Mother said that we could stay with them for about 1 month, but we needed to have our own home, and they would help Jonathan and me move to an apartment. My Dad has both dementia and Alzheimer, and it affects his short term. Jonathan and I agreed, and on August 3rd, I bought bus tickets for the 2 ½ days to Elmira.

I called my Mother as soon as we reached the bus station in Elmira, and it only took 10 minutes for her to drive there. She got out of the car and gave both of us a strong hug and she was excited to see me, but very excited to finally meet her grandson! We stopped at Burger King to buy a late Lunch, and arrived in Elmira around 3 p.m. My Dad helped carry our backpacks that contained our clothes.

I was worried that riding on the bus for 2 ½ days would cause me to have some nerve problems from sitting, but I did not. For me, being back in Elmira was not a big difference since I as already used to being in a big city of three million people compared to only about 60K in Elmira, but for Jonathan, this was a big transition having lived in Denver for his 21 years of life. He'd never even been out of Colorado, either.

It took Jonathan a couple months to transition, but Jonathan decided that he liked the small city.

August 28, 2015, we found an apartment we could afford, after about 3 weeks thanks to my Mother. It took us about a week, and we moved into our place on the third floor on August 28. But, would walking up and down the stairs daily, and leaving the apartment cause more problems? Surprisingly, it didn't, and I realized that walking up and down those three flights of stairs would affect me. However, to my shock, it actually made my muscles and nerves ache for about a week, but I was still using my cane. Jonathan did most of the walking up and down the steps, and my Mother helped when she could as well.

In January of 2016, I was diagnosed with Type 2 Diabetes. My Doctor said that this would affect with the healing of the nerve damage from the GBS. I found myself back in the hospital for three days to get my Blood sugar down from 380 to around 120. They did this by using high dose of insulin treatments four times a day. My pancreas was not producing insulin correctly.

By the summer of 2016, I was not using the cane at all. I still had some weak ankle muscles, but they were getting stronger, and I was able to control the ankles easier. The nerves were not yet totally healed. I also took a written driving test and passed. My Mother was my ride-along driver, and by November, I received my Driver's license. The last time I drove was just before going into the hospital in July 2006. It felt good driving again. I felt free.

As of now, December of 2018, the healing has yet to progress beyond my ankles. I'm beginning to believe that after 2 years, the nerves will never heal from the ankles to the toes. But, I have control over my ankles and some control in my toes. The doctor did say that the healing will be even slower for the nerve healing due to my diabetes.

Since most of what we do is on our feet a great amount of time, all I can do at this point is just watch what I do and how much. So far, thankfully, I have not had any Relapses.

My battle has been a very long road with GBS. Twelve, long years of emotional unrest, but I have fought, and I will continue to do so – one day at a time.

We will see, as time goes by, if the nerves will finally heal all the way to my toes.

Special Thanks To All

Rose Medical Center – Denver, Colorado

Neurologist
Dr. Machanic

And to all of the Doctors, Nurses, CNA's and the Social Services workers and all of the Physical /Occupational Therapists.

~~~~

Franklin Park Assistant Living Care Center - Denver, Colorado

To all of my Nurses, CNA's and the Social Services workers, the Physical Therapists, and of course the residents that I got to know, and all of the administrators and workers.

~~~~

Saint Joseph's Hospital - Elmira, New York

Physical Therapist
Cathleen Magee

Family Physician
Dr. Sosniak

Neurologist
Dr. Commins

www.ingramcontent.com/pod-product-compliance
Lightning Source LLC
Chambersburg PA
CBHW071117030426
42336CB00013BA/2124